Clinical Cases in Microbiology and Infectious Diseases

Clinical Cases in Microbiology and Infectious Diseases

Ghassan M. Matar, MSc, PhD
Professor and Vice Chairperson
Department of Experimental Pathology, Immunology, and Microbiology
Laboratory Director Center for Infectious Diseases Research (CIDR)
Faculty of Medicine
American University of Beirut
Lebanon

ELSEVIER

ELSEVIER

Elsevier

7th Circle, Zahran Plaza, 7th Floor, PO Box 140825, Amman, 11814, Jordan

Clinical Cases in Microbiology and Infectious Diseases, by Ghassan M. Matar

Copyright © 2017 Elsevier.

ISBN: 978-0-7020-7417-2
e-ISBN: 978-0-7020-7418-9

Content Strategist: Rasheed Roussan
Sr Project Manager—Education Solutions: Shabina Nasim
Content Development Specialist: Amani Bazzari
Project Manager: Nayagi Athmanathan
Cover Designer: Milind Majgaonkar

Printed in India

Contributors

Dania Abdallah, Pharm D
Pharmacy Department
Makassed General Hospital
Beirut, Lebanon

Rouba Abdennour, MD
Department of Pediatrics and Adolescent
Medicine
American University of Beirut
Beirut, Lebanon

Mohammad Abutaqa, MD
Division of Pediatric Cardiology
Department of Pediatrics and Adolescent
Medicine
Children's Heart Center
American University of Beirut
Beirut, Lebanon

Farah Al-Amin, MD
Division of Pediatric Infectious Diseases
Department of Pediatrics and Adolescent
Medicine
American University of Beirut
Beirut, Lebanon

Zainab Ali, MD
Department of Pediatrics and Adolescent
Medicine
Division of Pediatric Infectious Diseases
Center for Infectious Diseases Research
American University of Beirut
Beirut, Lebanon

Mariam Arab, MD
Division of Pediatric Cardiology
Department of Pediatrics and Adolescent
Medicine
Children's Heart Center
American University of Beirut
Beirut, Lebanon

George Araj, PhD
Center for Infectious Diseases Research
Department of Pathology and Laboratory
Medicine
American University of Beirut
Beirut, Lebanon

Aia Assaf-Casals, MD
Division of Pediatric Infectious Diseases
Department of Pediatrics and Adolescent
Medicine
American University of Beirut
Beirut, Lebanon

Lamya Atweh, MD
Department of Diagnostic Radiology
American University of Beirut
Beirut, Lebanon

Ali Bazarbachi, MD, PhD
Division of Hematology Oncology
Department of Internal Medicine
American University of Beirut
Beirut, Lebanon

Fadi Bitar, MD
Division of Pediatric Cardiology,
Department of Pediatrics and Adolescent
Medicine
Children's Heart Center
American University of Beirut
Beirut, Lebanon

Ahmad Chmaisse, MD
Center for Infectious Diseases Research
American University of Beirut
Beirut, Lebanon

Ibrahim Dabbous, MD
Department of Pediatrics and Adolescent
Medicine
American University of Beirut
Beirut, Lebanon

Ziad Daoud, PhD
Faculty of Medicine and Medical
Sciences
University of Balamand
Centre Hospitalier du Nord
Beirut, Lebanon

Ghassan Dbaibo, MD
Center for Infectious Diseases Research
Division of Pediatric Infectious Diseases
Department of Pediatrics and Adolescent
Medicine
Department of Biochemistry and
Molecular Genetics
American University of Beirut
Beirut, Lebanon

Soha Ghanem, MD
Department of Internal Medicine
Makassed General Hospital
Beirut, Lebanon

Christiane Haddad, MD
Department of Ophthalmology
American University of Beirut
Beirut, Lebanon

Rashid Haidar, MD
Division of Orthopedic surgery
Department of Surgery
American University of Beirut
Beirut, Lebanon

Hiba El Hajj, PhD
Department of Internal Medicine
Division of Hematology/Oncology
Department of Experimental Pathology,
Immunology and Microbiology
American University of Beirut
Beirut, Lebanon

Manal Hamdan, MD
Division of Infectious Diseases
Department of Internal Medicine
American University of Beirut
Beirut, Lebanon

Rima Hanna-Wakim, MD
Division of Pediatric Infectious Diseases
Department of Pediatrics and Adolescent
Medicine
Center for Infectious Diseases Research
American University of Beirut
Beirut, Lebanon

Souha S Kanj, MD
Division of Infectious Diseases
Department of Internal Medicine
American University of Beirut
Beirut, Lebanon

Roukoz Abou Karam, MS
Faculty of Medicine and Medical
Sciences
University of Balamand
Centre Hospitalier du Nord
Beirut, Lebanon

Joumana Kmeid, MD
Division of Infectious Diseases
Department of Internal Medicine
American University of Beirut
Beirut, Lebanon

Mona Koaik, MD
Department of Ophthalmology
American University of Beirut
Beirut, Lebanon

Dina Mahmassani, MD
Department of Internal Medicine
American University of Beirut
Beirut, Lebanon

Khalil Masri, MD
Centre Hospitalier du Nord
Beirut, Lebanon

Ghassan Matar, PhD
Center for Infectious Diseases Research
Department of Experimental Pathology,
Immunology, and Microbiology
American University of Beirut
Beirut, Lebanon

Habiba El Mchad, MD
Department of Internal Medicine
Makassed General Hospital
Beirut, Lebanon

Rima Moghnieh, MD
Department of Internal Medicine
Makassed General Hospital
Faculty of Medicine
Lebanese University
Beirut Arab University
Beirut, Lebanon

Salim Musallam, MD
Department of Pediatrics and Adolescent
Medicine
Division of Pediatric Infectious Diseases
American University of Beirut
Beirut, Lebanon

Mariam Rajab, MD
Department of Internal Medicine
Makassed General Hospital
Beirut, Lebanon

Issam Rassi, MD
Children's Heart Center
Department of Surgery
American University of Beirut
Beirut, Lebanon

Abdallah Rebeiz, MD
Department of Internal Medicine
Division of Cardiology
American University of Beirut
Beirut, Lebanon

Lina Reslan, PhD
Center for Infectious Diseases Research
American University of Beirut
Beirut, Lebanon

Nesrine Rizk, MD
Division of Infectious Diseases
Department of Internal Medicine
American University of Beirut
Beirut, Lebanon

Joseph Salameh, MD
Division of Neurosurgery
Department of Surgery
American University of Beirut
Beirut, Lebanon

Rida Salman, MD
Department of Diagnostic Radiology
American University of Beirut
Beirut, Lebanon

Rouba Shaker, MD
Division of Pediatric Infectious Diseases
Department of Pediatrics and Adolescent
Medicine
Center for Infectious Diseases Research
American University of Beirut
Beirut, Lebanon

Asem A. Shehabi, DSc
Department of Pathology and
Microbiology
The Jordan University
Amman, Jordan

Dania El Tabech, MD
Department of Internal Medicine
Makassed General Hospital
Beirut, Lebanon

Amer Toutonji, MD
Faculty of Medicine
American University of Beirut,
Beirut, Lebanon

Georges Zaytoun, MD
Department of Otolaryngology
American University of Beirut
Beirut, Lebanon

Zeinab El Zein, MD
Center for Infectious Diseases Research
American University of Beirut
Beirut, Lebanon

List of Reviewers

Isin Akyar, MD
Associate Professor
Microbiology Services Coordinator
Acibadem Labmed Medical Laboratories
Acibadem University School of Medicine, Dept of Medical Microbiology - Turkey

Yeşim Beşli, MD
Specialist in Medical Microbiology, Instructor
Acıbadem Labmed Clinical Laboratories, Microbiology Department,
Istanbul, Turkey
Acıbadem University Vocational School of Higher Education Health Sciences,
Istanbul, Turkey

Ziad Daoud, PhD
Professor of Clinical Microbiologist
Antimicrobial stewardship Consultant
Faculty of Medicine and Medical Sciences
University of Balamand, Lebanon

Asem A. Shehabi, PhD
Professor of Medical Microbiology
Faculty of Medicine, Department of Pathology-Microbiology
The Jordan University, Amman. Jordan

Sima Tokajian, PhD
Associate Professor of Microbial Genomics
Lebanese American University - Lebanon (LAU)

Foreword

It gives me great pleasure to write the foreword for *Clinical Cases in Microbiology and Infectious Diseases*, a publication of Elsevier, designed to accompany medical students in their years of training.

In recent years, we have witnessed an alarming surge in infectious diseases in terms of emergence of new pathogens as well as spread of new mechanisms of microbial resistance. Hospital- and community-acquired infections are becoming more difficult to treat, and this is creating a serious threat for public health at all levels. In this context, case discussion and analysis is one of the mainstays of the right diagnosis and appropriate patient management. Moreover, the use of clinical cases in problem-based learning has proven to be an efficient teaching approach for medical students.

The book *Clinical Cases in Microbiology and Infectious Diseases* consists of 13 chapters discussing different types of infections: bacterial, fungal, and parasitic. They describe excellent cases, some of which are very rarely reported, and constitute an exceptional opportunity for learning. All these chapters are instructive medical cases written in a professional way to "hold the students by the hand" and help them understand complex arguments.

This book constitutes an exciting and engaging read, not only for students but also for any doctor or health care professional interested in this field. The reader will find that the materials are structured in the most logical and helpful way and the chapters are fitted together for a better understanding of the text.

I congratulate the editor, Professor Ghassan Matar, for bringing out this wonderful book and appreciate the efforts put in by all the authors and contributors; they have done an excellent job. I am sure that the scientific, medical, and academic value of the material presented in this book is immense.

Ziad Daoud, PhD
Professor
Clinical Microbiology
Faculty of Medicine and Medical Sciences
University of Balamand, Beirut, Lebanon

Preface

With the emergence of new pathogens and the outbreaks that we are facing nowadays, infectious diseases persist worldwide among the prominent causes of mortality and morbidity. The effects of infectious diseases and their global spread prompts us to further investigate these diseases and the pathogens causing them in order to prevent their impact.

Clinical Cases in Microbiology and Infectious Diseases is an educational tool for students, researchers, and specialists, in which 12 medical cases are reported from hospitals across Lebanon; there is also an additional chapter that discusses the molecular methods for detection of common potentially sexually transmitted bacterial agents causing nonspecific urogenital infections.

The medical cases in this book tackle a wide range of pathogens and their clinical manifestations as reported by clinicians. Each chapter describes a medical case, with an overview, case presentation, examination, investigation, diagnosis, and treatment. At the end of each chapter, we have given a number of insightful questions that further enhances the understanding of the reported clinical case.

This book is based on clinical cases that were presented to three health care centers in Lebanon; nine cases from the American University of Beirut Medical Center, American University of Beirut, two cases from Makassed General Hospital, and one case from Balamand University Hospital. A descriptive chapter from Jordan University that discusses the molecular methods for detection of sexually transmitted bacterial agents is also included. Discussion of the cases would certainly empower medical students and specialists with the clinical manifestations of infections, their examination, and treatment.

Editor
Ghassan Matar

Acknowledgments

My deepest thanks go to ELSEVIER for inviting me to submit a book in the medical field, as well as to their team for facilitating the processing of the book.

I express my deep thanks to all the contributors of this book for devoting their time to report all the medical cases that they encountered. This book would not have been possible without their dedication and commitment.

Moreover, my sincere appreciation goes to Mr Sari S Rasheed for his assistance, comments, suggestions, and finalizing the book format.

Contents

Chapter 1

Bowel Perforation due to Methicillin-Sensitive Staphylococcal Enterocolitis in an Infant

Dania El Tabech, Soha Ghanem, and Mariam Rajab

ABSTRACT

In this report, we hereby present a case of a 3-month-old male infant with methicillin-sensitive staphylococcus aureus enteritis with small bowel perforation and bacteremia. The patient's signs and symptoms were typical of necrotizing enterocolitis with a surgical abdomen, even though the infant was neither in the typical age group nor was it the usual organism.

INTRODUCTION

Enterocolitis due to *Staphylococcus aureus* was first reported by Kramer in 1948 as a complication of treatment with antibiotics[1] and as arising in patients having predisposing conditions, such as previous treatment with a proton pump inhibitor, recent abdominal surgeries, and conditions compromising the immune system, such as immunosuppressive therapies, infection with HIV, and advanced age; and the culprit organism is usually methicillin-resistant *Staphylococcus aureus* (MRSA). Since the 1940s, sporadic cases and outbreaks were reported in infants, with low birthweight and prematurity being the main predisposing factors.

We hereby describe a 3-month-old baby boy, who developed a severe course of enteritis with small bowel perforation due to methicillin-sensitive *Staphylococcus aureus* (MSSA) with the source of transmission being due to bad hand hygiene from his caregiver's infected foot ulcer.

CASE

A three-month-old baby boy previously healthy, born by cesarean section (due to pre-eclampsia), full term, G1P1A0 with a birth weight of 3600 g, no delay in passage of meconium, received two doses of Hepatitis B, one dose of DTapHibIPV vaccines, formula fed, presented to Makassed General Hospital, a tertiary referral hospital in Lebanon, with the main complaint of 1 day of fever, irritability, and multiple episodes of nonbilious, nonprojectile vomiting without diarrhea or any other symptoms. Upon presentation, he had a temperature of 39°C, pulse 140, blood pressure 90/50 mm Hg, respiratory rate 38,

1

and oxygen saturation 100%. With regard to his anthropometric measurements, his height was at 75th percentile and weight at 95th percentile. He was conscious, irritable, ill looking, mildly pale, not in distress, had no bulging in anterior fontanel, clear chest, with a soft diffusely tender, mildly distended abdomen, and positive bowel sounds.

Full sepsis workup including lumbar puncture was done, and labs showed a WBC count of 15,600 with 5% bands, 86% neutrophils, C-reactive protein (CRP) 7.8; cerebrospinal fluid (CSF) analysis showed 20 RBCs/μL, 10 WBCs/μL (1 neutrophil and 9 lymphocytes), 73 mg/dL proteins, 54 mg/dL glucose; CSF and urine cultures were negative; and herpes and enterovirus detection by polymerase chain reactions (PCRs) in CSF were also negative.

On day 1 of hospitalization, vomiting stopped but the patient developed watery nonbloody diarrhea; stool studies done including microscopy, Rotavirus antigen detection, and culture were negative; the patient was tolerating PO intake but was still febrile and suffering with diarrhea, so treatment with gentamicin was started. Diarrhea continued until day 3 of hospitalization when his clinical condition deteriorated with redevelopment of vomiting, marked abdominal distention, and poor perfusion of the extremities. Hence, he was admitted to our pediatric intensive care unit and the antibiotics upgraded to vancomycin, meropenem, and metronidazole for broad spectrum coverage. CT scan of the abdomen showed marked distention of the bowel with pneumatosis intestinalis (Fig. 1.1).

In front of the surgical abdomen, exploratory laparotomy was done, which showed distended bowel loops with multiple small transverse lesions and one pinpoint small bowel perforation in the mid jejunal area (Figs. 1.2 and 1.3). Interrupted sutures were taken without bowel resection and culture taken from the peritoneal fluid grew MSSA; so did the blood culture that was taken on admission.

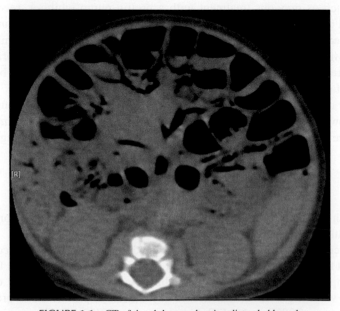

FIGURE 1.1   CT of the abdomen showing distended bowel.

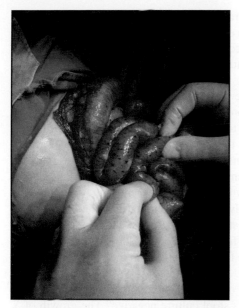

FIGURE 1.2 An intraoperative photograph showing distended small bowel with multiple small transverse lesions.

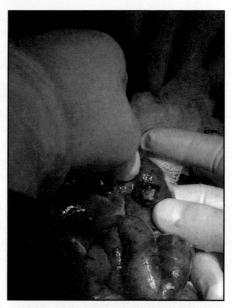

FIGURE 1.3 An intraoperative photograph showing friable jejunal area and a pinpoint perforation within.

Upon further history taking in an attempt to find the source of this organism, we found that the infant's caregiver had an infected ulcer on her ankle. A culture taken from the ulcer also grew MSSA with the same antibiotic sensitivity as in the infant's blood and peritoneal fluid.

DISCUSSION

Staphylococci are responsible for different gastrointestinal diseases, ranging from food poisoning to enterocolitis, as well as toxic shock syndrome in children[2] and adults.[3] *S. aureus* enteritis occurs mainly in adults and is usually antibiotic associated, postoperative, or occurs in cases of immunosuppression.[4,5] *S. aureus* enteritis rarely occurs in infants or toddlers; only a few cases are reported in the literature and almost all of them are antibiotic associated and due to MRSA.[6–8] In 1947, L. Selberg reported a case of *S. aureus* GI infection of an infant caused by his mother's staphylococcal mastitis.[6] In 1957, H.R. Morgan et al. reported a case of a 2.5-year-old female patient with staphylococcal enteritis with neither prior abdominal surgery nor recent antibiotic administration; however, unlike our case, the organism was a resistant *S. aureus*.[9] In March 1999, S.J. Han et al. described seven cases of infants, all younger than 3 months, who developed intestinal ulcerations and perforations intraoperatively similar to our patient but due to MRSA enteritis; moreover, most of the infants had a history of broad spectrum antibiotics consumption.[7] Only two of the seven infants survived. In April 1999, H. Kimata and M. Kawahara also reported MRSA enteritis in a 5-month-old immunocompetent infant with no predisposing factor.[8] However, our case describes enteritis with bowel perforation due to MSSA not MRSA.

A wide variety of toxins is produced by *S. aureus* strains that are responsible for disease pathogenesis. Toxic shock toxin (TSST-1), enterotoxin-like proteins, and staphylococcal enterotoxins are capable of functioning as superantigens having both systemic and local effects.[10] Different enterotoxins were identified in enterocolitis associated strains,[11] and they owe responsibility for the rise in erythrocyte sedimentation rates (ESR) and CRP level. Varying strains of *S. aureus* result in varying blends of toxins, hence the diversity in disease presentation.

Enterotoxins are produced in the lumen in the absence of tissue invasion, while inflammatory cells mostly are restricted to the lamina propria, thus implying that toxins can cross intact membranes.[12] Staphylococcal enterotoxins' toxic effects are mostly due to their impact on CD4+ T lymphocytes, although it was shown that epithelial cells may have toxin receptors (e.g. for TSST-1). Functioning as superantigens, staphylococcal enterotoxins are capable of activating lymphocytes independently of antigen specificity through binding MHC class II molecules and the T-cell receptor,[13] hence provoking cytokine secretion. Approximately 1:10,000 CD4+ T lymphocytes are normally involved in T-cell antigen stimulation; however, up to 50% of the T cells are stimulated by the staphylococcal superantigens producing a cytokine storm that affects both the structure and function of the intestine. The variability in specific superantigen binding is partly responsible for the difference in the severity of disease noticed throughout infections.[5,10,14]

The aforementioned facts explain the severity of the clinical picture of our patient; however, the question remains: why was our patient's stool culture negative? The growth of *S. aureus* in stool cultures is usually not reported by microbiology laboratories unless specifically requested, because it is one of the microbiologic floras normally inhabiting the gastrointestinal tract,[14,15] and because of the lack of guidelines that aid in determining the sufficient amount of *S. aureus* growth considered to be causing the diarrhea; hence, such cultures even when reported, require a cautious interpretation.[16]

CONCLUSION

Our case is unique and has not been previously described since the culprit organism is MSSA leading to enteritis with small bowel perforation in a 3-month-old infant acquired from the mother with an infected ulcer due to improper hand hygiene practice. Hence, *S. aureus*, even MSSA, should be considered in the differential diagnosis of a case of enteritis in infants, with emphasis on proper hand hygiene.

QUESTIONS

1. What are the common presentations of disease due to *Staphylococcus aureus*?
2. Explain the diversity observed in staphylococcal disease presentation.
3. In which type of patients has staphylococcal enterocolitis been previously described?
4. What are staphylococcal superantigens? How do they contribute to disease pathogenesis?
5. Why is the growth of *Staphylococcus aureus* in stool not commonly reported by microbiology laboratories?

REFERENCES

1. Kramer IRH. Fatal staphylococcal enteritis developing during streptomycin therapy by mouth. *Lancet.* 1948;1:646–651.
2. Gruber WC, Pietsch JB. Toxic shock syndrome associated with *Staphylococcus aureus* enterocolitis. *Pediatr Infect Dis J.* 1988;7(1):71–72.

3. Kotler DP, Sandkovsky U, Schlievert PM, et al. Toxic shock-like syndrome associated with staphylococcal enterocolitis in an HIV-infected man. *Clin Infect Dis.* 2007;44(12):e121–e123.

4. Iwata K, Doi A, Fukuchi T, et al. A systematic review for pursuing the presence of antibiotic associated entero-colitis caused by methicillin resistant *Staphylococcus aureus. BMC Infect Dis.* 2014;14(1):1.

5. Kotler DP, Sordillo EM. A case of *Staphylococcus aureus* enterocolitis: a rare entity. *Gastroenterol Hepatol.* 2010;6(2):117–119.

6. Selberg L. Fatal staphylococcal poisoning of a breast-fed infant whose mother suffered from staphylococcal mastitis. *Acta Obstet Gynecol Scand.* 1947;27(3):275–283.

7. Han SJ, Jung PM, Kim H, et al. Multiple intestinal ulcerations and perforations secondary to methicillin-resistant *Staphylococcus aureus* enteritis in infants. *J Pediatr Surg.* 1999;34(3):381–386.

8. Kimata H, Kawahara M. Methicillin-resistant *Staphylococcus aureus* enteritis in an immunologically uncom-promised infant. *Eur J Pediatr.* 1999;158(5):431–431.

9. Morgan HR, Breese BB, Greendyke RM. Primary staphylococcal enterocolitis. *AMA J Dis Child.* 1957; 93(5):526–529.

10. McCormick JK, Yarwood JM, Schlievert PM. Toxic shock syndrome and bacterial superantigens: an update. *Annu Rev Microbiol.* 2001;55(1):77–104.

11. Boyce JM, Havill NL. Nosocomial antibiotic-associated diarrhea associated with enterotoxin-producing strains of methicillin-resistant *Staphylococcus aureus. Am J Gastroenterol.* 2005;100(8):1828–1834.

12. Hamad AR, Marrack P, Kappler JW. Transcytosis of staphylococcal superantigen toxins. *J Exp Med.* 1997;185(8):1447–1454.

13. Li H, Llera A, Malchiodi EL, et al. The structural basis of T cell activation by superantigens. *Annu Rev Immunol.* 1999;17(1):435–466.

14. Kenneth T. *Staphylococcus aureus* and staphylococcal disease. In *Todar's Online Textbook of Bacteriology.* Madison, Wis, USA: University of Wisconsin-Madison Department of Bacteriology; 2008–2012.

15. Murray PR, Rosenthal KS, Pfaller MA. Commensal and pathogenic microbial flora in humans. In: Murray PR, Rosenthal KS, Pfaller MA, eds. *Medical Microbiology.* 5th ed. Philadelphia, PA: Elsevier Mosby; 2005:83–87.

16. Michael JT. *Staphylococcus aureus* enterocolitis: an underrecognized mimic of *Clostridium difficile. Infect Dis Clin Pract.* 2008;16(4):207–208.

Chapter 2

Orbital Cellulitis, Subperiosteal Abscess, Subdural Empyema, and Superior Sagittal Sinus Thrombosis: Intracranial Complications of Sinusitis Caused by *Streptococcus intermedius*

Rouba Shaker, Lina Reslan, Farah Al-Amin, Rida Salman, Lamya Atweh, Mona Koaik, Christiane Haddad, Georges Zaytoun, Joseph Salameh, George Araj, Ghassan M. Matar, and Ghassan Dbaibo

ABSTRACT

Sinusitis is a very common infection in children and adults. Complications of sinusitis can be serious and are particularly associated with frontal sinusitis. The etiology of intracranial or extracranial infections associated with sinusitis includes bacteria that commonly cause sinusitis, such as *Streptococcus pneumoniae* and *Haemophilus influenzae,* or other organisms that are less frequently associated with sinusitis, such as *Staphylococcus aureus* and anaerobes. In most cases, the responsible organism cannot be isolated due to the nature of these infections or because most patients would have received antibiotics prior to any interventional procedure. Here, we present a case of unilateral frontal sinusitis complicated by orbital cellulitis, subperiosteal abscess, subdural empyema, and superior sagittal sinus thrombosis where the responsible organisms *Streptococcus intermedius, Fusobacterium nucleatum,* and *Prevotella pleuritidis* were identified by the isolation and sequencing of 16S rDNA. The management of this and similar cases will be discussed in this chapter.

INTRODUCTION

Complications arising from rhinosinusitis are potentially life threatening and include venous sinus thrombosis, meningitis, and intracranial abscesses.[1] Diagnosis may be complicated by atypical presentations resulting in delayed treatment.[2] We encountered a rare combination of orbital cellulitis, subperiosteal abscess, subdural abscess, and superior sagittal sinus thrombosis following a late presentation of unilateral frontal sinusitis.

CASE REPORT

History and Presenting Symptoms

A 14-year-old male, previously healthy, presented with a 1-week history of fever and watery left eye discharge and a 3-day history of left upper eyelid edema, erythema, headache, and photophobia. Initially, he had used eye drops (ofloxacin and prednisolone), with no improvement. He was diagnosed as having periorbital cellulitis and was treated empirically with intramuscular ceftriaxone and oral amoxicillin–clavulanic acid 1 day prior to presentation. Prior to referral to our center, a computed tomography (CT) scan of the sinuses and orbits revealed opacification of the maxillary, ethmoidal, sphenoidal, and frontal sinuses on the left side with intraorbital abscess. The patient presented to our center for further workup and management.

Examination

On examination, it was found that he was febrile, drowsy, and sleepy. He had left frontal bossing with left eyelid erythema, swelling, and inability to open the left eye, which was almost closed. The neurological examination was significant for severe neck stiffness. On ophthalmological examination, the patient had mild left upper eyelid edema and tenderness with no associated duction deficit, and normal pupillary reactions. His vision was 20/20 in each eye with intraocular pressure of 15 mm Hg bilaterally; and he had no defect in eye motility or on fundoscopy.

Investigation

His C reactive protein level was 377 mg/L, and white cell count was 13300/mm^3. Cerebrospinal fluid (CSF) cell count revealed 4/mm^3 RBCs, 54/mm^3 WBCs with a differential of 73% neutrophils, 20% lymphocytes, 7% monocytes, with no detection of bacterial 16S ribosomal DNA (rDNA). Repeated CT of the brain with intravenous (i.v.) contrast revealed left pansinusitis and left subperiosteal collection overlying the left frontal bone (2.2 × 0.6 cm), small subperiosteal collection adjacent to the lamina papyracea with postseptal cellulitis, small left frontal subdural abscess extending medially to the level of the falx (1.4 × 0.6 cm), and a nonocclusive superior sagittal sinus (SSS) thrombus.

Diagnosis

Left pansinusitis with intracranial complications (left frontal subdural empyema), left frontal subperiosteal collection with postseptal cellulitis, and a nonocclusive SSS thrombus.

Management

He was started empirically on ceftriaxone, vancomycin, and metronidazole. Subcutaneous enoxaparin was initiated at a therapeutic dose for SSS thrombosis. Ceftriaxone and metronidazole were switched to ceftizoxime as he developed skin rash over the face and upper trunk after receiving metronidazole. The patient was followed up daily with subsequent resolution of his eyelid edema and decrease in left frontal swelling. Repeated CT of the brain with i.v. contrast showed improved SSS thrombosis and mild decrease in the size of the left epidural abscess. On day 5 of i.v. antibiotics, he developed a complex partial seizure lasting 10 min with eye deviation to the right and tonic movements of the upper extremities with loss of consciousness. Magnetic resonance imaging (MRI) of the brain showed intracranial extra-axial collection in the left frontal convexity reaching the anterior inferior falx cerebri that was increased in size compared to prior CT scans (Figs. 2.1 and 2.2). He underwent left intranasal endoscopic maxillary antrostomy, anterior and posterior ethmoidectomy, sphenoidotomy, frontal sinusotomy, and left frontal subperiosteal abscess incision and drainage. There was polyposis in all sinuses that were opened. Purulent discharge from sinuses and subperiosteal abscess was sent for culture and for bacterial 16S (rDNA) detection, amplification, and sequencing. Over the next 3 days, the patient continued to have fever and seizures. MRI of the brain with gadolinium showed slight interval increase in the left frontal subperiosteal abscess and the left frontal extra-axial abscess. Hence, he underwent left craniotomy and drainage of the subdural empyema 5 days following the sinus surgery (Fig. 2.3). Following surgery, the patient improved clinically, defervesced, and became free of seizures. Pus culture from the sinuses grew viridans streptococci, but culture from the left subperiosteal abscess and the subdural empyema did not show growth. The 16S rDNA polymerase chain reaction (PCR) result was positive for all specimens except the CSF. The sequence data were analyzed using BioEdit v7.2.5 software. All the sequences obtained were blasted using the BLAST (Basic Local Alignment Search Tool) server on the GenBank database at the National Center for Biotechnology Information (NCBI). These sequences were found to be consistent with *Streptococcus intermedius;* except for the subperiosteal specimen, the sequences showed two additional types of bacteria, *Fusobacterium nucleatum* and *Prevotella pleuritidis*. The

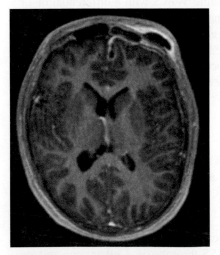

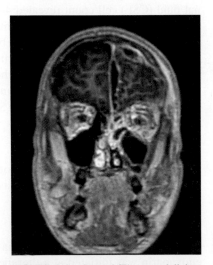

FIGURE 2.1   Axial T1 postgadolinium cut shows mucosal disease and enhancement of the left frontal sinus associated with extra-axial and subperiosteal abscesses. Abnormal enhancement of the left frontal bone is noted in keeping with osteomyelitis.

FIGURE 2.2   Coronal T1 postgadolinium cut shows leptomeningeal enhancement in the left fronto-parietal area and along the falx cerebri with an extra-axial abscess. Additional findings include osteomyelitis of the left frontal bone and mucosal disease.

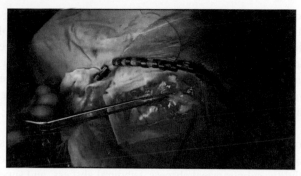

FIGURE 2.3   Intraoperative photo after the dura was incised to drain the left frontal subdural empyema.

latter sequence was analyzed on RipSeq Mixed Web application. This software has been used for direct 16S rRNA gene sequencing of clinical samples from polybacterial infections. The cultured viridans streptococcus minimum inhibitory concentration (MIC) for penicillin was 0.047. An allergy desensitization procedure for metronidazole was performed in order to optimize treatment for the three identified bacteria. The patient did not develop rash, and he was switched to penicillin and metronidazole. Repeated MRI venography of the brain showed no residual thrombosis in the cerebral venous sinuses. The thrombophilia workup was normal: antithrombin III 103 (N 83–128), lupus anticoagulant negative, protein C 78% (N 69–134), and protein S 94.5% (N 65–140), factor V activity 124.1% (N 52–138). His anticoagulation treatment was discontinued. The patient recovered well. He received a total of 20 days of i.v. antibiotics in the hospital and was discharged home to continue a total course of 6 weeks of i.v. antibiotics following the subdural empyema drainage.

Discussion

Intracranial complications have been reported in 10% of patients hospitalized with sinusitis.[3] These complications include meningitis, cavernous, and/or sagittal sinus thrombosis, epidural, subdural, and cerebral abscesses.[3] In children, periorbital cellulitis is the most common complication, followed by meningitis, intracranial abscess, and dural venous sinus thrombosis.[4] Patients commonly present with headaches (84%) and fevers (74%). Other findings include nausea and vomiting (38%), focal neurologic deficits (38%), mental status changes (32%), and seizures (18%). Forehead swelling, sinus tenderness, photophobia, lethargy, hemiparesis, and visual changes are less common signs and symptoms.[3] Only 28% of patients reported nasal symptoms of postnasal drip, nasal congestion, or rhinorrhea indicative of an acute sinusitis. Similarly, our patient presented with headache, photophobia, forehead swelling, left eyelid swelling, with no rhinorrhea or nasal congestion.

   MRI is considered more sensitive in diagnosing intracranial complications than CT, but it is poor at defining the bony anatomy required to plan endoscopic sinus surgery and can be difficult to do immediately.[5] Children older than 7 years, males, and those with neurologic status changes, frontal sinus opacification on CT, or the need for surgical intervention to drain an orbital abscess would benefit from MRI to rule intracranial extension.[6]

Simultaneous orbital and intracranial complications are rare following acute rhinosinusitis in pediatrics. In a study reported by Herrmann et al., the frequency of dual orbital and intracranial complications was 9.3% and this occurred only in children aged above 7 years.[6]

It is also considered rare to have multiple complications presenting in one patient.

A rare combination of periorbital cellulitis, subgaleal abscess, and superior sagittal sinus thrombosis following a late presentation of unilateral frontal sinusitis in a 14-year-old male patient was encountered.[2]

S. intermedius has been reported to be the cause of brain abscess in 18 patients in the pediatric population. However, only four of these cases were preceded by sinusitis.[7–10] Here, we report a case of a 14-year-old male patient presenting with multiple complications, including orbital cellulitis, subperiosteal abscess, subdural abscess, and superior sagittal sinus thrombosis arising from unilateral pansinusitis caused by *S. intermedius*.

Frontal sinuses are most commonly associated with sinogenic intracranial suppuration, followed in order by the ethmoid, sphenoid, and maxillary sinuses.[11] Frontal sinuses are poorly developed until the age of 10.[12] For this reason, it is believed that complications of pediatric sinusitis are relatively rare and mostly affect older children.[13] The odds ratio for developing intracranial complications is 20 if the frontal sinus is involved in the inflammatory process, compared to an odds ratio of 0.2 if the ethmoid sinus is involved.[13]

Intracranial extension of frontal sinusitis is thought to occur directly or by indirect hematogenous spread. Direct extension can progress by bacterial penetration of the posterior wall of the frontal sinus through necrotic areas of osteomyelitis. Retrograde extension of thrombophlebitis originating in the sinus mucosal veins can progress through the valveless diploic venous system (veins of Breschet) that interconnects the sinus mucosa to the meninges, skull and brain parenchyma, and dural venous sinuses.[14] Diploic veins are thin-walled, valveless veins lying in the diploe of the skull. In our patient, the polymicrobial infection from the left frontal sinusitis spread to cause orbital and periorbital cellulitis by direct extension. This likely progressed through the diploic and emissary veins resulting in a subperiosteal abscess overlying the left frontal bone from which *S. intermedius*, *F. nucleatum*, and *P. pleuritidis* were identified, small subperiosteal collection adjacent to the lamina papyracea with postseptal cellulitis, left frontal subdural empyema extending medially to the level of the falx, with a maximum thickness of 2 × 2 cm, and a nonocclusive SSS thrombus. It is postulated that infected emboli exacerbated the SSS thrombosis. Such emboli could potentially spread infection to more distant sites and this should always be considered while assessing similar cases.

As the patient received antibiotics prior to obtaining cultures from the sinuses, purulent drainage from the subdural empyema and from the subperiosteal abscess showed no growth, and only the pus drained from the sinuses grew viridans streptococci. However, the PCR result was positive for all specimens, identifying three different organisms. The 16S PCR has substantially enhanced the detection sensitivity for bacterial DNA in patient samples.[15] This highlights the importance of the use of bacterial 16S rDNA sequencing as a molecular diagnostic technique in the clinical microbiology laboratory to facilitate the diagnosis of infectious diseases of bacterial origin, especially in situations where samples are obtained after antibiotics have been administered, or where facultative organisms, or anaerobes are suspected.[15]

Although the sequencing from the subperiosteal abscess revealed three different types of bacteria including *S. intermedius*, *F. nucleatum*, and *P. pleuritidis*; only

S. intermedius was isolated from the subdural empyema. This is related to the bacterial virulence factors present in these bacteria, which constitute a part of the oropharyngeal flora.[16] *S. intermedius* is a member of the streptococcus anginosus group (SAG). It is a commensal of the gastrointestinal tract, but has the potential for significant morbidity.[17] *S. intermedius* possesses a group of surface proteins that are considered a major virulence factor termed antigen I/II that binds to human fibronectin and laminin, induces IL-8 release from monocytes, causing neutrophil chemotaxis, and activation.[17] The bacterium also has diverse protein antigens that contribute to apoptosis of specific lymphocyte subsets and suppress lymphocyte and fibroblast proliferation.[17] Another important virulence factor that some strains of *S. intermedius* possess is the polysaccharide capsule. The capsule allows the bacterium to escape phagocytosis, which, together with its biofilm formation ability, hinders the host immunity against it and allows it to replicate at the site of tissue damage.[17] The Streptococcus family also produces many hydrolytic enzymes including hyaluronidase, deoxyribonuclease, and chondroitin sulfatase that decrease tissue viscosity, allowing increased permeability and spread of infection through the liquefied tissue; they also work in synergy with anaerobic bacteria to cause tissue liquefaction and form abscesses.[17] Deutschman et al. showed that SAG associated infections were found to significantly cause neurological complications other than meningitis when compared to other bacteria causing rhinosinusitis ($P = .001$). These were also significantly more likely to induce permanent neurologic sequelae ($P = .02$).[18] Neurosurgical intervention was increasingly required in patients with SAG associated rhinosinusitis when compared to other bacteria (nine patients [64%] vs five [14%]; $P < .001$).[18] In addition, SAG associated infections required longer durations of i.v. antibiotic therapy compared with other bacteria (95% CI, 11–28 days; $t_{48} = 4.53$; $P < .001$).

Surgical incision and drainage combined with a long course of antibiotics (4–8 weeks) are the most common treatment modalities of an intracranial abscess complicating sinusitis.[3] The most common regimen of i.v. antibiotics was a long course of vancomycin, a third-generation cephalosporin, and metronidazole.[3] Similarly, our patient was started empirically on ceftriaxone, vancomycin, and metronidazole. Then, he was shifted to penicillin and metronidazole once the 16S identified the organisms involved and culture results showed susceptibility to penicillin.

The majority of patients with intracranial complications following acute sinusitis return to their baseline neurological status.[3] A minority of patients suffer permanent neurological sequelae, such as persistent seizures, hemiparesis, sensorineural hearing loss, and aphasia, especially in cases associated with delay in diagnosis, or delay in delivering appropriate treatment.[3] A study conducted by Germiller et al. found a favorable neurologic outcome, with only 8% long-term morbidity, and 4% mortality.[19] Our patient recovered completely and returned to his baseline neurological status with no postoperative symptoms.

CONCLUSION

Frontal sinusitis may be associated with potentially dangerous intracranial complications. Early diagnosis and treatment are essential to reduce morbidity, and mortality. Imaging plays an important role in the diagnosis of the disease and the detection of its complications. This case is one of the few reported cases of a rare combination of multiple complications of unilateral pansinusitis caused by *S. intermedius* in an immunocompetent child.

Management of these rare cases requires a multidisciplinary team, with early involvement of the radiologist, otolaryngologist, infectious diseases specialist, ophthalmologist, and neurosurgeon.

QUESTIONS

1. What are the major risk factors for intracranial complications of sinusitis?
2. Describe the mechanisms of intracranial extension of frontal sinusitis.
3. What is the gold standard of imaging modality for diagnosing intracranial complications of sinusitis?
4. Discuss the recommended treatment regimen for sinusitis with intracranial complications.
5. What are the major virulence factors that make *S. intermedius* an invasive pathogen?

REFERENCES

1. Patel AP, Masterson L, Deutsch CJ, Scoffings DJ, Fish BM. Management and outcomes in children with sinogenic intracranial abscesses. *Int J Pediatr Otorhinolaryngol*. 2015;79:868–873.
2. Jones H, Trinidade A, Jaberoo MC, Lyons M. Periorbital cellulitis, subgaleal abscess and superior sagittal sinus thrombosis: a rare combination of complications arising from unilateral frontal sinusitis. *J Laryngol Otol*. 2012;126:1281–1283.
3. Patel NA, Garber D, Hu S,Kamat A. Systematic review and case report: intracranial complications of pediatric sinusitis. *Int J Pediatr Otorhinolaryngol*. 2016;86:200–212.
4. Yeh CH, Chen WC, Lin MS, Huang HT, Chao SC, Lo YC. Intracranial brain abscess preceded by orbital cellulitis and sinusitis. *J Craniofac Surg*. 2010;21:934–936.
5. Younis RT, Anand VK, Davidson B. The role of computed tomography and magnetic resonance imaging in patients with sinusitis with complications. *Laryngoscope*. 2002;112:224–229.
6. Herrmann BW, Forsen JW, Jr. Simultaneous intracranial and orbital complications of acute rhinosinusitis in children. *Int J Pediatr Otorhinolaryngol*. 2004;68:619–625.
7. Brook I, Friedman EM. Intracranial complications of sinusitis in children. A sequela of periapical abscess. *Ann Otol Rhinol Laryngol*. 1982;91:41–43.
8. Tran MP, Caldwell-McMillan M, Khalife W, Young VB. Streptococcus intermedius causing infective endocarditis and abscesses: a report of three cases and review of the literature. *BMC Infect Dis*. 2008;8:154.
9. Yamamoto M, Fukushima T, Ohshiro S, et al. Brain abscess caused by Streptococcus intermedius: two case reports. *Surg Neurol*. 1999;51:219–222.
10. Onesimo R, Scalzone M, Valetini P, Caldarelli M. Pott's puffy tumour by *Streptococcus intermedius* a rare complication of sinusitis. *BMJ Case Rep*. 2011. doi: 10.1136/bcr.08.2011.4660.
11. Herrmann BW, Chung JC, Eisenbeis JF, Forsen JW, Jr. Intracranial complications of pediatric frontal rhinosinusitis. *Am J Rhinol*. 2006;20:320–324.
12. Adibelli ZH, Songu M, Adibelli H. Paranasal sinus development in children: a magnetic resonance imaging analysis. *Am J Rhinol Allergy*. 2011;25:30–35.
13. Hakim HE, Malik AC, Aronyk K, Ledi E, Bhargava R. The prevalence of intracranial complications in pediatric frontal sinusitis. *Int J Pediatr Otorhinolaryngol*. 2006;70:1383–1387.
14. Brook I. Microbiology and antimicrobial treatment of orbital and intracranial complications of sinusitis in children and their management. *Int J Pediatr Otorhinolaryngol*. 2009;73:1183–1186.
15. Sontakke S, Cadenas MB, Maggi RG, Diniz PP, Breitschwerdt EB. Use of broad range16S rDNA PCR in clinical microbiology. *J Microbiol Methods*. 2009;76:217–225.
16. Brook I. Microbiology and choice of antimicrobial therapy for acute sinusitis complicated by subperiosteal abscess in children. *Int J Pediatr Otorhinolaryngol*. 2016;84:21–26.

17. Mishra AK, Fournier PE. The role of *Streptococcus intermedius* in brain abscess. *Eur J Clin Microbiol Infect Dis*. 2013;32:477–483. Official publication of the European Society of Clinical Microbiology.
18. Deutschmann MW, Livingstone D, Cho JJ, Vanderkooi OG, Brookes JT. The significance of *Streptococcus anginosus* group in intracranial complications of pediatric rhinosinusitis. *JAMA Otolaryngol Head Neck Surg*. 2013;139:157–156.
19. Germiller JA, Monin DL, Sparano AM, Tom LW. Intracranial complications of sinusitis in children and adolescents and their outcomes. *Arch Otolaryngol Head Neck Surg*. 2006;132:969–976.

Chapter 3

Salmonella Osteomyelitis in a Healthy Child

Aia Assaf-Casals, Zeinab El Zein, Rouba Shaker, Rida Salman, Rima Hanna-Wakim, and Ghassan Dbaibo

ABSTRACT

We report a case of a 7-year-old, previously healthy girl, with salmonella osteomyelitis of the right distal fibula. The patient presented initially with limping and resolving low-grade fever with a history of trauma. Initial MRI results suggested traumatic injury; follow-up MRI done 1 month later revealed right distal fibular osteomyelitis. CT-guided biopsy was done and tissue was sent for culture, which grew *Salmonella* species. The patient received a total of 12 weeks of parenteral antibiotics. This is a rare case of salmonella osteomyelitis in a nonimmunocompromised, previously healthy patient.

INTRODUCTION

Acute osteomyelitis, a relatively common infection in developing countries, can be a devastating infection with serious sequelae if not treated early and promptly. Common organisms include *Staphylococcus aureus, Streptococcus pyogenes, Streptococcus pneumoniae, Kingella kingae,* and *Salmonella* species. In children, osteomyelitis due to *Salmonella* is uncommon and is typically associated with sickle cell disease, immunodeficiencies, malignancies, and other debilitating conditions.

CASE REPORT

History and Presenting Symptoms

A 7-year-old, previously healthy girl presented with a few days' history of right ankle swelling and low-grade fever; she was referred from the orthopedics department after magnetic resonance imaging (MRI) of the right ankle (Fig. 3.1A) showed diffuse bone marrow edema of the fibula with periosteal reaction, evidence of bone marrow contusion, and occult or trabecular fractures in keeping with a traumatic injury. Further history revealed that the patient had stayed with her grandmother who was admitted around 2 weeks before with *Salmonella* type C gastroenteritis. However, the patient herself had no history of gastroenteritis.

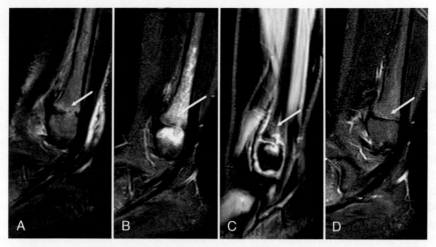

FIGURE 3.1   (A) Initial MRI of the ankle without gadolinium showing diffuse bone marrow edema of the fibula with periosteal reaction. Findings in keeping with a traumatic injury, bone marrow contusion, occult or trabecular fractures. No obvious fracture line could be identified. (B) MRI of the ankle with gadolinium after 1 month showing persistent bone marrow edema of the fibula with periosteal reaction and appearance of an enhancing 7 mm lesion in the distal fibular growth plate and extension into the lateral malleolus, consistent with progression of osteomyelitis. (C) MRI of the ankle with gadolinium. Comparison made with the previous MRIs shows that the described enhancing lesion at the level of the physis extending into the metaphysis and epiphysis (appearing lytic on CT) is grossly unchanged in size. However, it appears better defined with decrease in ill-defined enhancement; no typical liquefaction or abscess formation is seen yet. (D) MRI of the ankle with gadolinium showing resolution of the edema within the distal fibula. No enhancement post contrast administration. No evidence of fluid collections, fistulous tracts, or enhancing bone marrow edema in a manner to suggest osteomyelitis.

Examination

Initially, she was febrile with right ankle swelling. Shortly after admission, she became afebrile with resolution of her ankle swelling.

Investigation

Her inflammatory markers were only slightly elevated with a C-reactive protein (CRP) level of 4.9 mg/L, erythrocyte sedimentation rate (ESR) of 30 mm/h, and initial white blood cell (WBC) count of 8600 with 47% neutrophils. With a vague history of possible trauma, she was discharged home to repeat MRI in 2 weeks; however, MRI was not done until 1 month later. Meanwhile, evaluation in the clinic showed further decrease in inflammatory markers with a CRP level of less than 0.3 mg/L and ESR of 10 mm/h.

The follow-up MRI (Fig. 3.1B) revealed a right distal fibular 7 mm lytic lesion with periosteal reaction consistent with osteomyelitis in the absence of clinical symptoms. She was again admitted to the hospital and CT-guided biopsy of the lesion was done. Bone culture later grew *Salmonella* species not typeable with the available antisera; blood and stool cultures were negative. The inflammatory markers were persistently negative and the WBC count was still normal.

Diagnosis

Right distal fibular salmonella osteomyelitis with periosteal reaction.

Management

The patient was started on intravenous (i.v.) vancomycin and cefepime for empiric broad coverage of possible responsible pathogens. Bone culture later grew *Salmonella* species not typeable with the available antisera; blood and stool cultures were negative. A peripherally inserted central line (PICC) was placed and the patient was switched to i.v. ceftriaxone. Workup for possible immunodeficiency, including a dihydrorhodamine test to evaluate her for possible chronic granulomatous disease, was negative and no hemoglobinopathy was detected.

During her hospitalization, she developed abdominal pain and nausea. Biliary sludge was detected on ultrasound and she developed elevated transaminases. Hence, she was switched to cefotaxime for a total of 6 weeks. Follow-up MRI, however, showed that the previously described lytic lesion that extended into the metaphysis and epiphysis was grossly unchanged in size. Recognizing the indolent course of *Salmonella* organisms and the critical site of the lesion, a decision to continue out-patient intravenous cefotaxime for another 6 weeks was taken, since the follow-up MRI was still not reassuring (Fig. 3.1C).

The patient had a smooth course at home except for an allergic reaction to cefotaxime, for which she was switched to imipenem. Follow-up MRI at the end of treatment (Fig. 3.1D) showed significant improvement with complete resolution 6 months later. On follow-up, the patient is doing well with no evidence of sequelae or discrepancy in leg length.

DISCUSSION

Acute hematogenous osteomyelitis is the most common type of bone infection that occurs in children with a predilection for long bones, especially the femur.[1] The incidence varies between 1 and 13 per 100,000, with boys twice more affected than girls.[2] *S. aureus* is the most common causative pathogen followed by streptococcal and Gram-negative organisms. *S. pyogenes*, *K. kingae*, coagulase-negative staphylococci, and Enterobacteriaceae, such as *Escherichia coli*, *Klebsiella pneumoniae*, *Serratia marcescens*, and *Citrobacter* are less common causes.[1] *Salmonella*, mainly the nontyphoidal serotypes, has been identified as a frequent cause of osteomyelitis in children with sickle cell disease or immunosuppression. There are about 2600 serotypes of *Salmonella enterica* infections that usually present as gastroenteritis, enteric fever, bacteremia with or without focus, and asymptomatic carriage.[3,4] *Salmonella* is rarely a cause of osteomyelitis in healthy children. Only 24 cases of salmonella osteomyelitis in healthy children have been reported from 1978 to 2014.[4–7] Here we report a new case of salmonella osteomyelitis in an otherwise healthy child. There was no history of recent gastroenteritis to suggest a source for hematogenous spread to the bone, although a subclinical infection with transient bacteremia may have led to the seeding of the bone, which may have been injured previously by unrecalled trauma. In most of the previously reported cases, the infection was mainly in long bones followed by pelvic bones. Similarly, our patient had osteomyelitis of the right distal fibula. Interestingly, the patient had very subtle symptoms and low to absent inflammatory markers as compared to previous reports of cases presenting with elevated inflammatory markers.[5,8] This suggests that some *Salmonella* serotypes may evade the immune response causing only a transient elevation of inflammatory markers that might be missed. The ability to enter host cells, particularly phagocytes, is an essential feature in the pathogenesis of *Salmonella*. After entering into host cells, *Salmonella* undergoes transformation and induces immune modulation in order to replicate and disseminate without being identified by the host's immune system.[9,10] Signaling kinases, other enzymes, and pro-inflammatory transcription factors are targeted to manipulate and suppress host cellular immune responses including AvrA acetyltransferase, MAPK kinases, NFκB, and JNK.[10,11] These abilities could explain why inflammatory markers may remain within the normal range as noticed in the current case. In more than half of the cases, MRI or CT was initially done and provided a high diagnostic yield of osteomyelitis compared to other modalities.[8] However, in the current case, the initial MRI suggested traumatic injury only, possibly due to a very early presentation before the complete picture evolved. After 1 month, the follow-up MRI revealed right distal fibular lesion with periosteal reaction consistent with osteomyelitis. As for the treatment, most of the patients in the previous papers received ampicillin or third-generation cephalosporins for a total duration of 4–6 weeks.[3–5,8] In a few of the reported cases, the patient had to undergo surgical debridement or drainage. Some experts recommend the use of vancomycin or clindamycin for empiric treatment of osteomyelitis in communities with greater than 10% of the community acquired methicillin-resistant *S. aureus*, with vancomycin being preferred in communities with clindamycin resistance rates of more than 25%.[11] Once *Salmonella* species is isolated, targeted therapy includes third-generation cephalosporins or fluoroquinolones.[3] Focal infections caused by *Salmonella* should be drained or debrided whenever possible. In a normal host with a surgically eradicated focus, it is suggested that antimicrobial therapy is continued for a minimum of 4–6 weeks.[1,2] Salmonella osteomyelitis is usually difficult to treat. Quinolone resistance has been emerging and failure of fluoroquinolones demonstrated.[12] As for our patient, she received a total of 12 weeks of parenteral antibiotics with no surgical intervention. The duration of treatment was prolonged because the first follow-up MRI was not reassuring. Follow-up MRI 6 months after the end of treatment, however, showed complete resolution of osteomyelitis.

CONCLUSION

Knowing the indolent course of *Salmonella* infections in general and osteomyelitis in particular, *Salmonella* species should be suspected and targeted even in otherwise healthy children when presenting with an exceptionally "cold" osteomyelitis. A high index of suspicion is necessary in order to pursue microbiological diagnosis necessary to optimize the choice of treatment and its duration.

QUESTIONS

1. What are the most common causative organisms of osteomyelitis in children?
2. List three conditions that increase the risk of salmonella osteomyelitis and mention how to diagnose them.
3. What is the best imaging modality for diagnosis of osteomyelitis and for its follow-up?
4. What is the empiric treatment of osteomyelitis, especially salmonella osteomyelitis?
5. What is the role of surgery in the management of salmonella osteomyelitis?

REFERENCES

1. Conrad DA. Acute hematogenous osteomyelitis. *Pediatr Rev.* 2010;31(11):464–471.
2. Yeo A, Ramachandran M. Acute haematogenous osteomyelitis in children. *BMJ* 2014;348:g66.
3. McAnearney S, McCall D. Salmonella osteomyelitis. *Ulster Med J.* 2015;84(3):171–172.
4. Saturveithan C, Arieff A, Premganesh G, et al. Salmonella osteomyelitis in a one year old child without sickle cell disease: a case report. *Malays Orthop J.* 2014;8(2):52–54.
5. Tsagris V, Vliora C, Mihelarakis I, et al. Salmonella osteomyelitis in previously healthy children: report of 4 cases and review of the literature. *Pediatr Infect Dis J.* 2016;35(1):116–117.
6. Sipahioglu S, Askar H, Zehir S. Bilateral acute tibial osteomyelitis in a patient without an underlying disease: a case report. *J Med Case Rep.* 2014;8:388.
7. Adeyokunnu AA, Hendrickse RG. Salmonella osteomyelitis in childhood. A report of 63 cases seen in Nigerian children of whom 57 had sickle cell anaemia. *Arch Dis Child.* 1980;55(3):175–184.
8. Matono T, Takeshita N, Kutsuna S, et al. Indolent non-typhoidal salmonella vertebral osteomyelitis in a diabetic patient. *Intern Med.* 2015;54(23):3083–3086.
9. Broz P, Ohlson MB, Monack DM. Innate immune response to *Salmonella typhimurium*, a model enteric pathogen. *Gut Microbes* 2012;3(2):62–70.
10. Velge P, Wiedemann A, Rosselin M, et al. Multiplicity of *Salmonella* entry mechanisms, a new paradigm for *Salmonella* pathogenesis. *Microbiology Open* 2012;1(3):243–258.
11. Harik NS, Smeltzer MS. Management of acute hematogenous osteomyelitis in children. *Expert Rev Anti-infect Ther.* 2010;8(2):175-81.
12. Hohmann EL. Nontyphoidal salmonellosis. *Clin Infect Dis.* 2001;32(2):263–269.

Chapter 4

An Adolescent with an Unusual Presentation of Neurobrucellosis

Rouba Abdennour, Aia Assaf-Casals, Rima Hanna-Wakim, Rouba Shaker, Rida Salman, George Araj, and Ghassan Dbaibo

ABSTRACT

Brucellosis is one of the most common zoonotic infections worldwide with high prevalence in the Mediterranean and Middle Eastern countries. It is a multisystem disease with a broad clinical spectrum ranging from asymptomatic infection to severe or even fatal infection. Neurological involvement has been reported in up to 7.6% of patients with brucellosis. Diagnosis of neurobrucellosis can be problematic, as no definite diagnostic criteria have been set so far. In this report, we describe a 17-year-old male who presented with an acute onset of altered level of consciousness and vomiting, and a 6-month history of headache, nausea, episodes of vomiting, and fatigue. He was diagnosed with neurobrucellosis based on brucella indirect (CAPT) titers turned of $\geq$1:1280 in blood and 1:320 in CSF. The patient had initially responded well to treatment with antituberculous medications that included rifampin and amikacin before the diagnosis of neurobrucellosis was confirmed and he was switched to doxycycline, rifampin, and amikacin. Neurobrucellosis presents with nonspecific manifestations that may mimic several pathologies making diagnosis challenging. Thus, a high index of suspicion should be kept, especially in culture negative meningitis/encephalitis with subacute presentation. Despite the fact that systemic brucellosis is commonly encountered in the region, neurobrucellosis remains an uncommon manifestation, and to the best of our knowledge, this is the first report of an adolescent with neurobrucellosis in Lebanon.

INTRODUCTION

Brucellosis is one of the most common zoonotic infections worldwide with high prevalence in the Mediterranean and Middle Eastern countries. It is a multisystem disease with a broad clinical spectrum ranging from asymptomatic to severe or even fatal infection.[1] Neurological involvement has been reported in around 2%– 7.6% of cases with brucellosis.[2,3] Diagnosis of neurobrucellosis can be problematic as no definite diagnostic criteria have been set so far.

CASE PRESENTATION

A 17-year-old adolescent male presented to the emergency department (ED) with a 2-day history of vomiting, altered level of consciousness, and slurred speech.

The parents also reported a 6-month history of occasional nausea and vomiting, headache, weight loss, decreased activity, and weakness. He had no fever, cough, or sick contacts.

19

EXAMINATION

In the ED, he was agitated and sleepy. He was disoriented, not following commands, and his physical exam was pertinent for positive meningeal signs.

INVESTIGATION

MRI of the brain revealed high Fluid Attenuated Inversion Recovery (FLAIR) signal, diffusion restriction, and enhancement of the cerebrospinal fluid (CSF) cisterns and sulci consistent with meningitis (Fig. 4.1A and B).

CT angiography of the head was normal with no evidence of venous sinus thrombosis. Blood work showed a white blood cell (WBC) count of 12,300/mm^3 with 86% lymphocytes, hemoglobin of 12.6 g/dL, platelets of 224,000/mm^3, and inflammatory markers within the normal range. CSF analysis revealed CSF pleocytosis with lymphocyte predominance (WBC 206/mm^3 with 78% lymphocytes), low glucose of 12 mg/dL, and an elevated protein level of 5.37 g/L. Vancomycin, ceftriaxone, and acyclovir were initiated for empiric treatment of meningitis. Polymerase chain reaction (PCR) for enteroviruses and herpes simplex virus (HSV) were negative in the CSF and bacterial CSF culture showed no growth. Workup for tuberculosis (TB) infection showed a nonreactive Purified Protein Derivative (PPD), a negative interferon-gamma release assay (IGRA), no acid-fast bacilli in the sputum, negative *Mycobacterium tuberculosis* PCR in the CSF, and clear lungs on X-ray and CT of the chest. Despite the laboratory results, tuberculous meningitis was highly suspected because of the subacute presentation and negative bacterial cultures, and the patient was started on anti-TB therapy with 4-drug regimen (rifampin, isoniazid, ethambutol, and pyrazinamide) in addition to amikacin and dexamethasone. Screening of the family members showed that a 22-year-old brother had a reactive PPD but a clear chest X-ray. Shortly thereafter, his clinical symptoms improved with no residual neurologic deficits. Magnetic resonance imaging (MRI) of the brain was repeated and revealed significant resolution of the previously present brain abnormalities with persistent enhancement at the level of the quadrigeminal cistern (Fig. 4.2A and B).

Brucella titers came back after initiation of anti-TB therapy showing serum brucella direct titer <1:20 and indirect titer ≥1:1280, and in the CSF, brucella direct titer <1:20 and indirect titer 1:320.

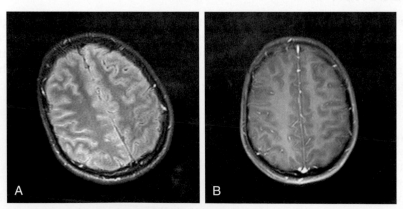

FIGURE 4.1 (A) MRI of the brain upon admission: High FLAIR signal, diffusion restriction, and enhancement of the CSF cisterns and sulci. (B) B is another view.

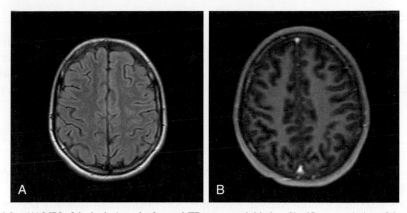

FIGURE 4.2   (A) MRI of the brain 1 week after anti-TB treatment initiation: Significant resolution of the previously present brain abnormalities with persistent enhancement at the level of the quadrigeminal cistern. (B) B is another view.

DIAGNOSIS

Neurobrucellosis

MANAGEMENT

Doxycycline was added to his treatment. All CSF bacterial, fungal, and mycobacterial cultures were negative; therefore, anti-TB therapy was discontinued but he was maintained on rifampin and completed a 4-week course of amikacin. His follow-up CSF studies, 2 months into treatment showed improved glucose and protein levels, but a slightly increased CSF leukocyte count compared to the previous CSF analysis as shown in Table 4.1. Eight months later, the patient is doing well, free of symptoms, continuing rifampin and doxycycline, and is being followed up with Lumbar punctures (LPs) until normalization of CSF studies and brucella titers (Table 4.1).

TABLE 4.1 Serial Cerebrospinal Fluid Analyses Results

Day of Admission	RBC (/mm³)	WBC (/mm³)	Lymphocytes (%)	Glucose (mg/dL)	Protein (g/L)	Brucella Indirect[a]
Day 0	9	206	78	12	5.37	-
Day 1	21	162	70	23	4.06	-
Day 12	30	277	98	13	3.4	-
Day 25	277	0	0	22	2.25	1:320
3 months later	0	56	97	41	1.17	1:160
7 months later	2	14	95	47	0.58	1:80

RBC, red blood cell; WBC, white blood cell.
[a]All brucella direct titers were <1:20.

DISCUSSION

Chronic meningitis has a wide differential diagnosis with multiple potential causative infectious agents, including bacteria, viruses, fungi, mycobacteria, and parasites. Chronic meningitis may also be secondary to noninfectious etiologies, such as neoplasms, sarcoidosis, or drug-induced. An etiology may not be identified in up to one-third of all patients even with an extensive workup.[4]

CLINICAL PRESENTATION

Brucellosis is highly prevalent in the Mediterranean countries, South and Central America, Eastern Europe, Asia, Africa, the Caribbean, and the Middle East.[5]

Reports state that Central Nervous System (CNS) involvement typically occurs in 3%–5% of patients with brucellosis[6] and may reach up to 7.6%[2]; however, given the heterogeneity of its clinical manifestations and the delays in diagnosis, the incidence of neurobrucellosis might be higher. For instance, meningeal irritation only occurs in one-third of the patients, and findings that are frequently seen in systemic brucellosis such as hepatosplenomegaly are rarely present in patients with CNS involvement. Neurological involvement in brucellosis can present as acute or chronic meningitis, encephalitis, myelitis, radiculitis, and/or neuritis involving cranial or peripheral nerves. The cranial nerves (CN) most commonly involved are the eighth leading to sensorineural hearing loss, and the sixth resulting in abducens palsy. Brucellar CN palsies usually resolve with antibiotics, whereas chronic CNS infection may result in permanent neurologic deficits.[5] Neurobrucellosis may also cause vasculitis affecting any vascular structure, and can manifest as either the rupture of a mycotic aneurysm or arteritis resulting in lacunar infarcts, small hemorrhages, or venous thrombosis.[7]

DIAGNOSIS

This case illustrates the importance of establishing a diagnosis in cases of chronic meningitis. Our primary suspicion in this regard was TB meningitis on the basis of clinical presentation and the reactive PPD in the brother. However, the lack of confirmatory test results led us to investigate the etiology further despite the marked clinical improvement with anti-TB treatment. In retrospect, this was due to the overlapping effectiveness of rifampin and amikacin against both TB and brucella. The use of dexamethasone likely contributed to the rapid clinical improvement before doxycycline was added. Serologic assays in addition to regular cultures are the most commonly used tests in the diagnosis of brucellosis.[8] IgM first appears after contracting the infection followed by IgG within 10–14 days. These titers decline slowly during the recovery phase. Persistently elevated titers indicate poor response to treatment.[9] For unknown reasons, serum antibodies (mainly IgG and some IgM) may persist for months/years in up to 15%–20% of asymptomatic patients who have undergone treatment and cure.[10] Serum agglutination tests (SAT) are fairly simple, sensitive, provide rapid results, and are reliable for acute infection. However, they have a high rate of false-negatives in chronic brucellosis, in which case indirect Coombs is the preferred method. Brucellacapt has a similar sensitivity to Coombs test but is done in a single step and can detect the nonagglutinating IgG and IgA antibodies. Enzyme immunoassay (EIA) and/or Brucellacapt are the tests of choice for complicated and chronic cases and are able to detect Ig classes and subclasses. However, in order to have an accurate diagnosis, combination tests are preferred: the serum agglutination test (SAT) and the brucella indirect Coombs test, SAT and Brucellacapt, or SAT and the enzyme-linked immunosorbent assay (ELISA).[11] In acute brucellosis, these tests show elevated levels of IgG, IgM, IgA, IgE, IgG1, and IgG3, whereas in chronic brucellosis, an elevation in IgG, IgA, IgE, IgG1, and IgG4 has been observed. In relapsed cases, there is an increase in IgG and IgA, but not in IgM.[9] If highly suspected, brucellosis should not be excluded even if titers are negative, since some *Brucella* subclasses and early disease may yield false-negative results.[11] In patients with chronic neurobrucellosis, Gram-stain and cultures in the CSF, and blood are often negative and poorly sensitive[5]. However, CSF in these patients contains low titers of antibodies.[12] In a study by Lulu et al. of 25 patients with neurobrucellosis, ELISA was positive for IgG in all patients, IgM in 16%, and IgA in 88%.[10] Both direct and indirect brucella titers should be taken because direct titers may be falsely negative and miss the diagnosis, as in our patient.

Other diagnostic tests include molecular assays such as conventional polymerase chain reaction assay (PCR) and real-time PCR, but these need standardization and optimization.[11]

Imaging findings in neurobrucellosis have been classified into four types: normal, abnormal enhancement indicating enhancement, white matter changes on T2, and vascular changes. White matter changes may mimic other inflammatory or infectious diseases, such as multiple sclerosis, acute disseminated encephalomyelitis, or Lyme disease.[13,14]

With all these testing methods in mind, there are no definite diagnostic criteria for neurobrucellosis yet. Criteria commonly used are: the presence of any neurological sign or symptom, CSF lymphocytic pleocytosis, elevated protein, and low glucose levels in the CSF, with isolation of *Brucella* from blood or CSF, or positive SAT or Coombs or presence of *Brucella* antibodies in CSF at any titer.[15,16] Teke et al. also include MRI or CT findings in the diagnostic criteria.[16]

TREATMENT

There are three factors to take into consideration while selecting the best antibiotics for treating neurobrucellosis. *Brucella* replicates intracellularly without affecting the cellular cycle and bacterial load may be present in apparently healthy individuals for years after the infection; it has a high rate of relapse, and antibiotics should have the capacity to cross the blood–brain barrier. Therefore, a prolonged course with a combination of 2–3 drugs is required.[17] Streptomycin is almost always a part of the combination treatment and has been more recently replaced by gentamicin because of its easier administration.[17] Trimethoprim–sulfamethoxazole (TMP–SMX) and rifampicin can cross the blood–brain barrier and achieve therapeutic CSF levels and should always be part of the treatment regimen, since aminoglycosides and tetracyclines have poor penetration to the CSF. According to the 2006 WHO recommendations, rifampin or TMP–SMX should always be added to the standard regimen of doxycycline plus streptomycin.[19] Though aminoglycoside-based regimens have been shown to have higher efficacy, rifampin–doxycyline combination has been more popularly used because of its easier administration and fewer side effects.[17] Another additional agent could be ceftriaxone. Treatment with ceftriaxone is usually started upon presentation for any patient presenting with a picture of meningitis or encephalitis before the diagnosis of neurobrucellosis is made, and it may allow shorter treatment course.[6] All this would explain the clinical improvement in our patient after initiating anti-TB treatment, which included rifampin and amikacin. Children below 8 years of age with brucellosis should be treated with oral TMP–SMX for at least 6 weeks with a parenteral aminoglycoside for the first 14 days of therapy. For children 8 years and above, doxycycline for at least 6 weeks in addition to streptomycin for 3 weeks or gentamicin for the first 10–14 days are the gold standard of treatment.[17,18] Rifampin may be added to further decrease the risk of relapse.[20]

There are no randomized controlled trials on the duration of therapy in neurobrucellosis. Treatment is generally prolonged over several months, not less than 3 months; it needs to be individualized and should be continued until CSF parameters have normalized. Steroids may be used in cases complicated by iritis, papilledema, myelopathy, polyneuropathy, and/or cranial nerve palsy.[10]

Outcomes

An inverse relationship exists between the duration of symptoms and outcome. Mortality secondary to neurobrucellosis is rare, ranging from 0% to 5.5%, but some clinical sequelae such as sensorineural hearing loss may be permanent. In addition, many patients experience vague neuropsychiatric symptoms or chronic fatigue-like symptoms even after achieving complete cure, suggesting a possible alteration of biochemical parameters at the subcellular level.[6,15]

CONCLUSION

In conclusion, neurobrucellosis presents with nonspecific manifestations that may mimic several pathologies making the diagnosis challenging. Thus, a high index of suspicion should be kept, especially in patients with subacute presentation and culture-negative meningitis/encephalitis.

QUESTIONS

1. How does neurobrucellosis present?
2. What are the best available diagnostic criteria for neurobrucellosis?
3. What is the differential diagnosis of chronic meningitis?
4. What is the optimal treatment regimen of neurobrucellosis and its duration in children over 8 years? In children under 8 years?
5. What is the outcome of neurobrucellosis?

REFERENCES

1. Colmenero JD, Reguera JM, Martos F, et al. Complications associated with *Brucella melitensis* infection: a study of 530 cases. *Medicine.* 1996;75(4):195–211.
2. Bosilkovski M, Krteva L, Dimzova M, Kondova I. Brucellosis in 418 patients from the Balkan Peninsula: exposure-related differences in clinical manifestations, laboratory test results, and therapy outcome. *Int J Infect Dis.* 2007;11(4): 342–347.
3. Doganay M, Aygen B. Human brucellosis: an overview. *Int J Infect Dis.* 2003;7:173.
4. Sexton DJ. Chronic meningitis. In: Calderwood SB, ed. *UpToDate.* The Netherlands: Wolters Kluwer; 2015. Accessed 17.08.16.
5. Gul HC, Erdem H, Bek S. Overview of neurobrucellosis: a pooled analysis of 187 cases. *Int J Infect Dis.* 2009;13(6):e339–e343.
6. Pappas G, Akritidis N, Christou L. Treatment of neurobrucellosis: what is known and what remains to be answered. *Expert Rev Anti Infect Ther.* 2007;5(6):983–990.

7. Adaletli I, Albayram S, Gurses B, et al. Vasculopathic changes in the cerebral arterial system with neurobrucellosis. *Am J Neuroradiol.* 2006;27(2):384–386.
8. Araj GF. Update on laboratory diagnosis of human brucellosis. *Int J Antimicrob Agents.* 2010;36(Suppl 1): S12–S17.
9. Araj G. Brucella. In: Jorgensen J, Pfaller M, Carroll K, Funke G, Landry M, Richter S, Warnock D, eds. *Manual of Clinical Microbiology.* 11th ed. Washington, DC: SM Press; 2015:863–872.
10. Lulu AR, Araj GF, Khateeb MI, Mustafa MY, Yusuf AR, Fenech FF. Human brucellosis in Kuwait: a prospective study of 400 cases. *Q J Med.* 1988;66(249):39–54.
11. Araj G. Standard and New Laboratory Procedures in neurobrucellosis. In: Turgut M, Haddad FS, de Divitiis O, eds. *Neurobrucellosis: Clinical, Diagnostic and Therapeutic Features.* Switzerland: Springer International Publishing AG; 2016:143–148.
12. Erdem H, Kilic S, Sener B, et al. Diagnosis of chronic brucellar meningitis and meningoencephalitis: the results of the Istanbul-2 study. *Clin Microbiol Infect.* 2013;19(2):E80–E86.
13. Ceran N, Turkoglu R, Erdem I, et al. Neurobrucellosis: clinical, diagnostic, therapeutic features and outcome. Unusual clinical presentations in an endemic region. *Braz J Infect Dis.* 2011;15(1):52–59.
14. Jiao LD, Chu CB, Kumar CJ, et al. Clinical and laboratory findings of nonacute neurobrucellosis. *Chin Med J.* 2015;128(13):1831–1833.
15. Karsen H, Tekin koruk S, Duygu F, Yapici K, Kati M. Review of 17 cases of neurobrucellosis: clinical manifestations, diagnosis, and management. *Arch Iran Med.* 2012;15(8):491–494.
16. Teke TA, Koyuncu H, Oz FN, et al. Neurobrucellosis in children: case series from Turkey. *Pediatr Int.* 2015;57(4):578–581.
17. Cerván A, Hirschfeld M, Rodriguez M, Guerado E. Medical therapy of neurobrucellosis. In: Turgut M, Haddad FS, de Divitiis O, eds. *Neurobrucellosis: Clinical, Diagnostic and Therapeutic Features.* Switzerland: Springer International Publishing AG; 2016:151–159.
18. Ulu-kilic A, Karakas A, Erdem H, et al. Update on treatment options for spinal brucellosis. *Clin Microbiol Infect.* 2014;20(2):O75–O82.
19. Corbel M. Treatment of uncomplicated brucellosis in adults and children eight years of age and older. In: *Brucellosis in humans and animals.* Geneva: World Health Organization; 2016:36–41. Accessed 24.08.16.
20. Bosilkovski M. Clinical manifestations, diagnosis, and treatment of brucellosis. In: Calderwood SB, Edwards MS, eds. *UpToDate.* The Netherlands: Wolters Kluwer; 2016. Accessed 17.08.16.

Chapter 5

Salmonella enterica Serovar Paratyphi B Subdural Empyema in a Child with Malaria

Zainab Ali, Rouba Shaker, Aia Assaf-Casals, Zeinab El Zein, Rida Salman, Salim Musallam, Ibrahim Dabbous, and Ghassan Dbaibo

ABSTRACT

A 5-year-old male patient presented to the emergency department with signs and symptoms of increased intracranial pressure in the setting of acute falciparum malaria infection. Upon undergoing imaging, drainage, and culture, he was found to have *Salmonella enterica* serovar Paratyphi B subdural empyema. Subdural empyema has been reported in the literature in two patients with *Plasmodium falciparum* infection. Since both infections are endemic in many countries, their coinfection of the same host is likely. The occurrence of subdural empyema in a patient with malaria should prompt the consideration of *Salmonella* as a possible agent.

INTRODUCTION

Malaria remains the world's major infectious disease, causing a high death rate among affected people compared to other infectious diseases.[1,2] Globally, *Plasmodium falciparum* is the most important species responsible for causing severe malaria as well as cerebral malaria.[2] Association of subdural empyema and malaria is very rare. There are only two reported cases of spontaneous subdural empyema in available literature.[3,4] To our knowledge, there are no reported cases of *Salmonella* causing subdural empyema in the setting of malaria. Here we present a rare and interesting case of falciparum malaria that is complicated by subdural empyema induced by *Salmonella enterica* serovar Paratyphi B.

CASE REPORT

History and Presenting Symptoms

A 5-year-old Lebanese boy, residing in Liberia, West Africa, with a history of West Syndrome and recurrent malarial infections, presented to the emergency department at the American University of Beirut Medical Center (AUBMC) with severe headache and progressive hypoactivity of 5 days' duration. Ten days prior to presentation, he had developed high-grade fever reaching 40°C with vomiting. Malaria smear performed in Liberia showed

Plasmodium falciparum with high parasitemia (more than 3%). Accordingly, he received artemether and ceftriaxone injections in Liberia for 3 days, and then continued on oral mefloquine.

However, the patient had a poor response to treatment and became progressively more lethargic over the next few days prompting his family to fly him to AUBMC in Beirut, Lebanon.

Examination

He was afebrile with a normal respiratory rate and bradycardia (56 beats/min). He was pale, agitated, and drowsy. The abdomen was soft with mild splenomegaly. There were negative meningeal signs and no focal neurological deficit. All reflexes were preserved with intact sensory and motor functions.

Investigation

The patient underwent general investigations including blood count, electrolytes, and liver enzymes. He was found to have anemia with low hemoglobin of 10.2 g/dL, slightly elevated white blood cell (WBC) count of 15,200/mm^3 with 78% neutrophils, and a platelet count of 90,000/mm^3. The rest of the laboratory tests were normal. The repeated malaria test, done in Liberia, prior to his presentation to AUBMC, turned out to be positive for *P. falciparum*. ECG showed sinus bradycardia. Malaria thin and thick smear done at AUBMC were negative. Blood, urine, and stool cultures were negative. In the context of bradycardia, headache, and agitation, brain computed tomography (CT) scan was performed to rule out increased intracranial pressure. Unexpectedly, the scan showed a right hemispheric subdural collection with a maximum thickness of 3 cm, causing significant mass effect on the surrounding brain parenchyma, with midline shift of 2 cm and subfalcine herniation (Fig. 5.1A).

A right parietal burr hole and evacuation of the right hemispheric subdural collection were performed. The subdural fluid was purulent; it was sent for analysis and culture. The analysis showed glucose <3 mg/dL, protein 43 g/L, RBC 70,000/mm^3, and WBC count of 1100/mm^3 with 99% neutrophils. The culture grew *S. enterica* serovar Paratyphi B.

Since the presentation was unusual, immune workup was performed. HIV serology, IgE level quantitation of CD4, CD8, and CD19 cell counts and dihydrorhodamine test were all within normal limits. The histopathology of the brain and dural membrane did not reveal any evidence of parasitic malaria infection.

Diagnosis

Cerebral malaria complicated with *S. enterica* serovar Paratyphi B subdural empyema.

Management

Subsequently, the patient received 7 days of treatment with intravenous (i.v.) quinine and clindamycin in addition to 6 weeks i.v. ceftriaxone. Repeated CT brain in 2 months showed significant decrease in the right cerebral subdural collection mainly along the right temporal lobe associated with thickening of the dura at this level measuring 1 cm at its maximal transverse diameter (previously 2 cm), with decrease in the shift of the midline to the left

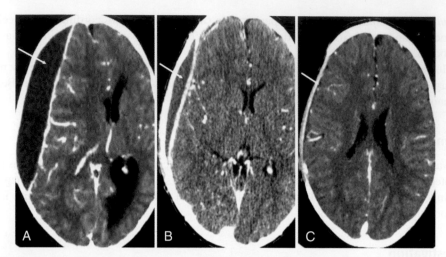

FIGURE 5.1 (A) Initial enhanced CT showing right hemispheric subdural collection (arrow) with enhancement of the surrounding dura and few thin septation, causing significant mass effect and brain herniation. (B) Enhanced CT, 2 months after right parietal burr hole and antibiotic treatment showing decrease in the size of the right-sided subdural fluid collection (arrow) with associated mass effect on the right hemisphere. (C) Enhanced CT, 5 months after initial CT showing resolution of the subdural empyema (arrow).

measuring 5.5 mm (previously 9 mm) (Fig. 5.1B). Repeated CT of the brain in 5 months showed interval resolution of the subdural empyema (Fig. 5.1C).

DISCUSSION

Severe malaria is defined as acute malaria with signs of organ dysfunction and/or high level of parasitemia (more than 4%–5% infected erythrocytes or more than 250,000 parasites/µL).[5] Cerebral malaria is a severe neurological complication of malaria and has an incidence of 120/100,000 per year in endemic areas of Africa. It is defined by the WHO as a clinical syndrome characterized by coma at least 1 h after termination of a seizure or correction of hypoglycemia, asexual forms of *P. falciparum* parasites on peripheral blood smears, and no other cause to explain the coma.[6,7] However, recent reports suggest that the rate of severe malaria is decreasing.[8–10] Severe malaria occurs in 1% of patients infected with *P. falciparum*.[11]

The presence of distinct strains of the parasites in a given geographical area and the existence of antigenic variation during the infection force the host to mount immune response against these different strains and antigenic variants. Moreover, in the absence of reinfection with malaria for about 6 months to 1 year, the previously developed antimalarial immunity starts to wane. Therefore, the short-lived immunity acquired against malaria is species- and strain-specific.[12]

This is illustrated by our patient, who despite living in Liberia, where malaria is endemic, had two previous malarial infections, with the third encounter being the most severe despite his intact immunity. However, the most likely explanation for the severity of this third episode was the coinfection with *S. enterica* serovar Paratyphi B and *P. falciparum*.

Focal lesions in malaria are infrequent with subdural empyema being very rare. There have been two case reports of subdural empyema with *P. falciparum* in the literature. The first was reported by Huda et al.,[4] where a 70-year-old male who had been treated for falciparum malaria 7 days before, presented to the emergency department in altered sensorium and later developed right-sided hemiparesis. Noncontrast CT revealed left-sided frontoparietal subdural hematoma with subfalcine and transtentorial herniation. A craniotomy was done to evacuate the hematoma. He received i.v. artisunate and antibiotics. Few days postoperatively, the patient started to regain the ability to localize painful stimuli and open his eyes spontaneously; however, he passed away secondary to aspiration pneumonia.[4]

A second case was reported by Dwarakanath et al.,[3] where a 3-year-old girl presented unconscious after a seizure while on antimalarial treatment. A left hemispheric subdural hematoma with mass effect and midline shift was detected by a noncontrast CT. Fungal, regular, and TB cultures of the purulent Cerebrospinal Fluid (CSF) obtained upon surgical evacuation were negative. Histopathology from intraoperative tissue did not show any malarial parasite. Postoperatively, the child was maintained on i.v. quinine and ceftriaxone, amikacin, and metronidazole. Although she started to improve postoperatively, 2 weeks later she died after she developed chest infection, bacterial meningitis, and septicemia.

The diagnosis of Cerebral Malaria (CM) is based on the clinical presentation of cerebral dysfunction and blood smear tests.[13] Imaging may show cerebral edema (thalamic and white matter hypodensities on CT, and focal or diffuse T2-hyperintense lesions on MRI), cortical or subcortical strokes, and multiple microbleeds.[13]

CM may also be seen on ophthalmoscopy as patchy retinal whitening, focal changes of vessel color, or retinal bleeding.[14] We hypothesize that the vasculopathy observed in CM played a role in the pathogenesis of the *S. enterica* serovar Paratyphi subdural collection in this case. The patient may have acquired *S. enterica* serovar Paratyphi from the community, developed a bacteremia, and seeded the subdural space. Whether there was a preexisting collection induced by malaria in this space prior to *S. enterica* serovar Paratyphi infection cannot be determined. Also, the neurological findings that led to the initial diagnosis of CM in our patient could have also been caused by the purulent collection infected with *S. enterica* serovar Paratyphi. The coexistence of these two rare conditions in this patient with a normal immune function favors the pathogenetic link that we proposed.

The treatment of choice of cerebral malaria in sub-Saharan Africa is quinine.[15] However, a recent study on 5000 African children with CM showed that those taking artesunate had better outcome and recommended that artesunate should replace quinine in the treatment of cerebral malaria.[15] Despite the proper management with artemether and mefloquine that were administered initially, our patient continued to have neurological deterioration likely induced by the *S. enterica* serovar Paratyphi collection that was discovered later. Consequently, i.v. quinine and clindamycin were given for 7 days. In addition, he received i.v. ceftriaxone for a total of 6 weeks as a treatment for *S. enterica* serovar Paratyphi coinfection.

CONCLUSION

Fatal and distressing complications can be expected in patients with CM. Bacterial coinfection should be considered in unusual course of recovery during the treatment of malarial infection using appropriate medications. Additionally, patients with intact immune system may not get protected from the hazardous effect of *P. falciparum*. This is the first case report of a spontaneous subdural empyema complicating CM from which *S. enterica* serovar Paratyphi B was cultured. It highlights a serious complication that is likely to be encountered, since these two organisms are endemic in the same regions raising the need for adequate imaging in atypical presentations.

QUESTIONS

1. What are the diagnostic criteria for cerebral malaria?
2. How common is subdural empyema in malaria?
3. What is the best approach for the treatment of subdural empyema?
4. What is the optimal treatment for cerebral malaria?
5. What is the definition of severe malaria?

REFERENCES

1. Snow RW, Omumbo JA, Lowe B, et al. Relation between severe malaria morbidity in children and level of *Plasmodium falciparum* transmission in Africa. *Lancet.* 1997;349(9066):1650–1654.
2. Gay F, Zougbede S, N'Dilimabaka N, Rebollo A, Mazier D, Moreno A. Cerebral malaria: what is known and what is on research. *Revue Neurol.* 2012;168(3):239–256.
3. Dwarakanath S, Suri A, Mahapatra AK. Spontaneous subdural empyema in falciparum malaria: a case study. *J Vector Borne Dis.* 2004;41(3-4):80–82.
4. Huda MF, Kamali NI, Srivastava VK, Kaif M. Spontaneous acute subdural hematoma in malaria: a case report. *J Vector Borne Dis.* 2011;48(4):247–248.
5. Crawley J, Chu C, Mtove G, Nosten F. Malaria in children. *Lancet.* 2010;375(9724):1468–1481.
6. Idro R, Marsh K, John CC, Newton CR. Cerebral malaria: mechanisms of brain injury and strategies for improved neurocognitive outcome. *Pediatr Res.* 2010;68(4):267–274.
7. Baird JK. Severe and fatal vivax malaria challenges 'benign tertian malaria' dogma. *Ann Trop Paediatr.* 2009;29(4):251–252.
8. Okiro EA, Hay SI, Gikandi PW, et al. The decline in paediatric malaria admissions on the coast of Kenya. *Malar J.* 2007;6:151.
9. Nyarango PM, Gebremeskel T, Mebrahtu G, et al. A steep decline of malaria morbidity and mortality trends in Eritrea between 2000 and 2004: the effect of combination of control methods. *Malar J.* 2006;5:33.
10. Garg RK. Cerebral malaria. *J Assoc Physicians India.* 2000;48(10):1004–1013.
11. Snow RW, Guerra CA, Noor AM, Myint HY, Hay SI. The global distribution of clinical episodes of *Plasmodium falciparum* malaria. *Nature.* 2005;434(7030):214–217.
12. Doolan DL, Dobano C, Baird JK. Acquired immunity to malaria. *Clin Microbiol Rev.* 2009;22(1):13–36.
13. Abdel Razek AA, Watcharakorn A, Castillo M. Parasitic diseases of the central nervous system. *Neuroimaging Clin N Am.* 2011;21(4):815–841, viii.
14. Molyneux EM, Mankhambo LA, Phiri A, et al. The outcome of non-typhoidal salmonella meningitis in Malawian children, 1997-2006. *Ann Trop Paediatr.* 2009;29(1):13–22.
15. Dondorp A, Nosten F, Stepniewska K, Day N, White N, South East Asian Quinine Artesunate Malaria Trial g. Artesunate versus quinine for treatment of severe falciparum malaria: a randomised trial. *Lancet.* 2005;366(9487):717–725.

Chapter 6

Mycobacterium fortuitum Bacteremia and Pneumonia in a Child with T-Cell Lymphoma Presenting with Febrile Neutropenia

Rouba Shaker, Ahmad Chmaisse, Aia Assaf-Casals, George Araj, Salim Musallam, Ghassan Dbaibo, and Rima Hanna-Wakim

ABSTRACT

Rapidly growing mycobacteria (RGM) are a group of nontuberculous mycobacteria (NTM) that usually grow in subculture within one week. RGM include three clinically relevant species: *Mycobacterium fortuitum*, *Mycobacterium chelonae*, and *Mycobacterium abscessus*. Exposure to these organisms, which are widely distributed in water and soil, may lead to superficial and invasive infections. These microorganisms cause a wide spectrum of clinical syndromes in both immunocompetent and immunocompromised hosts, including osteomyelitis, respiratory tract, bloodstream, and disseminated infections. *M. fortuitum* is the most commonly encountered species of this group isolated from nonrespiratory specimens. We report a case of *M. fortuitum* bacteremia with pneumonia in a 2-year-old child with T-cell lymphoma presenting with febrile neutropenia.

INTRODUCTION

Among the genus *Mycobacterium*, rapidly growing mycobacteria (RGM) are considered to account for almost half of the entire species. Their ability to grow macroscopic colonies in less than 7 days,[1] along with their ability to develop biofilms, have made some of the RGM clinically relevant in both immunocompetent and immunocompromised patients.[2,3,4] These disease-causing mycobacteria have been associated with surgical sites, posttraumatic wounds, disseminated skin and soft tissue infections, bones, joints, lungs, and other sites of infections.[5] Of these strains, the three most common are *Mycobacterium fortuitum*, *M. chelonae*, and *M. abscessus*.[6] Furthermore, some studies on the prevalence of these mycobacteria in cancer patients have shown the lungs to be the most commonly affected organs in immunocompromised individuals; more common in adults than in children.[7,8] To our knowledge, this is the first case of RGM NTM central venous catheter (CVC)-related bloodstream infection with dissemination to the lungs in a pediatric cancer patient to be reported in our region.

CASE REPORT

History and Presenting Symptoms

A 2-year-old male patient, diagnosed with T-cell lymphoma, 7 months prior to presentation, on maintenance chemotherapy, presented to the hospital with febrile neutropenia; he had a 1-day history of fever reaching 38.4°C, along with a dry cough. His recent chemotherapy was 3 weeks prior to admission. He was started on empiric broad spectrum antibiotics with intravenous cefepime and vancomycin.

Examination

Aside from some petechial lesions found on the patient's scalp and oral mucosa, clinical examination was unremarkable.

Investigation

Laboratory investigations showed a WBC count of 500/mm^3, absolute neutrophil count of zero, and a platelet count of 20,000/mm^3. Blood culture from the central line grew NTM after 89 h. Computed tomography (CT) of the neck, abdomen, and pelvis revealed no abnormalities. CT of the chest, on the other hand, revealed patches of ground-glass abnormalities in the right lung field, and pulmonary nodules showing the "halo sign" consistent with mycobacterial infection in both lungs.

Diagnosis

Mycobacterium fortuitum bacteremia and pneumonia.

Management

He was started initially on triple antibiotic therapy consisting of amikacin, rifampin, and azithromycin pending susceptibility testing, and his CVC was removed. Speciation testing done at Mayo Medical Laboratories (Rochester, MN, USA) confirmed the presence of *M. fortuitum*. The susceptibility testing revealed that the isolate was susceptible to trimethoprim–sulfamethoxazole (TMP–SMX), linezolid, imipenem, ciprofloxacin, moxifloxacin, and amikacin. The mycobacterium was resistant to clarithromycin, tobramycin, and doxycycline. Inducible clarithromycin resistance through erythromycin methylase (erm) gene was detected.

Follow-up CT of the chest, after 3 months of treatment, revealed resolution of many of the previously seen bilateral lung nodules, with persistence of three nodules in the right lung. After the susceptibility results, the antimycobacterial treatment regimen was changed to oral TMP–SMX and ciprofloxacin to continue a total course of 12 months. Almost 6 months after the initial bacteremia and pulmonary nodules, no appreciable lung nodules were detected on CT of the chest.

DISCUSSION

Despite their low virulence and mortality rate, RGM's ability to create biofilms has made them possible sources of infections in CVCs.[9] RGM bacteremia, although rare, is encountered in immunocompromised hosts, especially in cancer patients.[10] The most common underlying malignancies are hematologic in nature[9]; cancers affecting lymphocytes, specifically, disrupt their ability to fight mycobacterial infections[11].

In a 10-year retrospective study,[8] three distinct syndromes were identified in cancer patients with RGM infections: the most common was pulmonary disease, which occurred in 47% of the patients; bloodstream infections, affecting 45% of the patients; and disseminated infections, occurring in 8% of the patients. *M. fortuitum* bacteremia has also been implicated with sternal wound infection, disseminated disease, prosthetic valve endocarditis, and intravascular catheter cellulitis.[12]

The current case describing a child diagnosed with T-cell lymphoma who developed *M. fortuitum* bacteremia that disseminated to the lungs is one of only a few cases of similar infections reported in this age group. The neutropenia present in our patient is a major risk factor for RGM infections although they have also been observed in patients without neutropenia.

In the treatment of RGM infections, several important issues must be taken into account. These include: avoiding monotherapy in severe infections due to the possibility of acquiring resistance, checking for the presence of foreign material on which biofilms may have formed (e.g., prosthetic valves, catheters, pacemakers), and determining the nature of the infection.[1] Removing the foreign material, such as the CVC in the current and other reported cases,[10,11] becomes an urgent and integral part of treatment. In a study by Chang CY et al.,[10] timely catheter removal was able to decrease the possibility of relapsing bacteremia from 75% in patients with delayed catheter removal to zero in those with timely catheter removal.

Several studies have shown resistance of *M. fortuitum*, *M. chelonae*, and *M. abscessus* to first-line antituberculous drugs, such as streptomycin, isoniazid, rifampicin, ethambutol, and ethionamide.[1,11,13,14] Second-line antituberculous drugs, aminoglycosides and quinolones, are more effective against these RGM strains.[1,13]

Specifically, *M. fortuitum* has been shown to be susceptible to aminoglycoside antibiotics, such as amikacin, capreomycin, kanamycin, and tobramycin. Other effective antibiotics include: tigecycline, linezolid, cefmetazole, macrolides, moxifloxacin, TMP–SMX, and carbapenems.[1,13] Similarly, our patient was started empirically on amikacin, rifampin, and azithromycin. Susceptibility testing also revealed that the *M. fortuitum* isolate was susceptible to linezolid, imipenem, ciprofloxacin, moxifloxacin, and amikacin. Following this, he was shifted to TMP–SMX and ciprofloxacin to continue a total course of 12 months. The inducible clarithromycin resistance, described by some reports to be related to the erm (39) gene,[13] was also detected in our case. Therefore, selecting a proper therapeutic scheme for RGM infections requires an *in vitro* susceptibility test of the individual strain.[1]

CONCLUSION

RGM are important pathogens in biofilm-related infections; mainly catheter-related bloodstream infections. These bloodstream infections have been reported in patients with cancer [7]. Catheter removal and treatment with an effective combination of antimycobacterial drugs is necessary.[1,11,15] Most of the RGM species are susceptible to amikacin; this agent may be considered in the initial empiric treatment regimen of RGM bacteremia.[1,13,14] The duration of therapy depends upon the site and severity of infection as well as the host's immune status.[15]

QUESTIONS

1. What are the major predisposing factors for mycobacterial infections?
2. What makes RGMs more clinically relevant than other NTMs?
3. What are the common clinical syndromes associated with RGM infections?
4. Before initiating therapy for RGM infections, what are some important considerations to take into account?
5. What combination therapies are optimal in the empirical treatment of NTMs?

REFERENCES

1. Esteban J, Ortiz-Perez A. Current treatment of atypical mycobacteriosis. *Expert Opin Pharmacother.* 2009;10(17):2787–2799.
2. Tagashira Y, Kozai Y, Yamasa H, et al. A cluster of central line-associated bloodstream infections due to rapidly growing nontuberculous mycobacteria in patients with hematologic disorders at a Japanese tertiary care center: an outbreak investigation and review of the literature. *Infect Control Hosp Epidemiol.* 2015;36(1):76–80.
3. Henkle E, Winthrop KL. Nontuberculous mycobacteria infections in immunosuppressed hosts. *Clin Chest Med.* 2015;36(1):91–99.
4. Dailloux M, Abalain ML, Laurain C, et al. Respiratory infections associated with nontuberculous mycobacteria in non-HIV patients. *Eur Respir J.* 2006;28(6):1211–1215.
5. Hawkins C, Qi C, Warren J, et al. Catheter-related bloodstream infections caused by rapidly growing nontuberculous mycobacteria: a case series including rare species. *Diagn Microbiol Infect Dis.* 2008;61(2):187–191.
6. Fernandez-Roblas R, Esteban J, Cabria F, et al. In vitro susceptibilities of rapidly growing mycobacteria to telithromycin (HMR 3647) and seven other antimicrobials. *Antimicrob Agents Chemother.* 2000;44(1):181–182.
7. Apiwattankul N, Flynn PM, Hayden RT, et al. Infections caused by rapidly growing *Mycobacteria spp* in children and adolescents with cancer. *J Pediatric Infect Dis Soc.* 2015;4(2):104–113.
8. Redelman-Sidi G, Sepkowitz KA. Rapidly growing mycobacteria infection in patients with cancer. *Clinic Infect Dis.* 2010;51(4):422–434.
9. Rathor N, Khillan V, Panda D. Catheter associated mycobacteremia: opening new fronts in infection control. *Indian J Crit Care Med.* 2015;19(6):350–352.
10. Chang CY, Tsay RW, Lin LC, et al. Venous catheter-associated bacteremia caused by rapidly growing mycobacteria at a medical center in central Taiwan. *J Microbiol, Immunol Infect [Wei Mian Yu Gan Ran Za Zhi].* 2009;42(4):343–350.
11. Zainal Muttakin AR, Tan AM. *Mycobacterium fortuitum* catheter-related sepsis in acute leukaemia. *Singapore Med J.* 2006;47(6):543–545.
12. Hoy JF, Rolston KV, Hopfer RL, et al. *Mycobacterium fortuitum* bacteremia in patients with cancer and long-term venous catheters. *Am J Med.* 1987;83(2):213–217.
13. Pang H, Li G, Zhao X, et al. Drug susceptibility testing of 31 antimicrobial agents on rapidly growing Mycobacteria isolates from China. *BioMed Res Int.* 2015;2015:419392.
14. Makarova MV, Freiman GE. [Study of the drug-sensitivity of nontuberculous mycobacteria]. *Tuberk Bolezni Legkikh.* 2009(7):55–58.
15. Piersimoni C, Scarparo C. Extrapulmonary infections associated with nontuberculous mycobacteria in immunocompetent persons. *Emerg Infect Dis.* 2009;15(9):1351–1358; quiz 544.

Chapter 7

Acute Osteomyelitis with *Ureaplasma urealyticum* Following an Infected Hydrocele Resection in a Lymphoma Patient on Maintenance Rituximab

Joumana Kmeid, Nesrine Rizk, Rashid Haidar, Ali Bazarbachi, and Souha S. Kanj

ABSTRACT

The following case is of a 40-year-old man known to have non-Hodgkin follicular lymphoma on rituximab, presenting with clinical and radiological evidence of right ankle septic arthritis and osteomyelitis, 1 week after treatment of an infected hydrocele.

The standard bacterial, mycobacterial, and fungal cultures were repeatedly negative, and the patient's condition progressively worsened despite broad-spectrum antibiotic coverage.

The patient underwent surgical debridement and molecular testing using the 16S ribosomal RNA polymerase chain reaction, which turned positive identifying *Ureaplasma urealyticum*.

U. urealyticum, a nonvirulent pathogen, has been associated with serious infection, such as osteomyelitis and septic arthritis depending on the host's immune status.

CASE PRESENTATION

This is the case of a 40-year-old man who presented on April 20, 2013, with the chief complaint of right ankle pain of 4-day duration.

The patient reported that his ankle pain was associated with swelling and warmth of the joint and redness of the overlying skin. These symptoms were progressing and limiting the patient's ability to walk. No fever was documented; however, chills were reported.

The patient was diagnosed with a non-Hodgkin follicular lymphoma in 2011. At that time, he received a chemotherapy regimen consisting of cyclophosphamide, doxorubicin, vincristine, and prednisone plus rituximab. Then he was maintained on rituximab administered every 2 months; last dose received 1 day prior to presentation.

On April 16, 2013, the patient underwent surgical excision of a right hydrocele. No intraoperative cultures were taken; however, the patient was discharged on an unknown antibiotic for a presumed infected hydrocele. The patient denied any previous sexually transmitted diseases, but reported unprotected heterosexual activity with multiple partners.

Other than his ankle pain, the patient reported only minimal dysuria on review of systems.

Examination

His physical examination was notable for right ankle edema, erythema, and warmth of the overlying skin. Joint effusion with marked limitation of active and passive ranges of motion and tenderness were noted. All other joints were normal. No skin abnormalities were seen except around the right ankle. Genital examination showed no erythema, no effusion, and nontender smooth right testis; there was no discharge around the surgical site and no other abnormal findings in the scrotal and perianal areas.

Investigation

Laboratory work-up was as follows: WBC count 8900 cells/mm^3 with 73% polymorphonuclear cells and 19% lymphocytes; hemoglobin 12.8 g/dL; normal platelets, creatinine, uric acid, and electrolytes. A joint fluid aspiration performed on admission revealed: WBC count 64,000/mm^3 with 88% polymorphonuclear cells; no crystals; negative cultures after 5 days of incubation; negative *Chlamydia trachomatis* DNA-PCR and negative *Neisseria gonorrhea* DNA-PCR. Results of urine polymerase chain reactions (PCRs) for *C. trachomatis* and *N. gonorrhea* were also negative. Furthermore, the following test results were negative: HIV 1 and 2 antibodies and P24 antigen; HBsAg; VDRL-RPR qualitative; Brucella direct and indirect Coombs. The patient was started on cefepime and vancomycin; he received 3 days of intravenous antibiotics, improved clinically and was discharged on ceftriaxone, 1 g daily for a total of 14 days and doxycycline, 100 mg twice daily for 7 days. A repeat ankle fluid aspiration performed on May 7, 2013, showed a WBC count of 15,680/mm^3 with 88% polymorphonuclear cells and a negative culture. After this partial improvement, the patient presented again to American University of Beirut Medical Center (AUBMC) on June 19, 2013, with a gradual worsening of his right ankle pain, worsening of the erythema, and a new skin lesion overlying the joint that appeared after using a herbal cream. There was no documented fever. Physical examination showed significant swelling and erythema over the medial and lateral aspects of the right ankle with bullous formation of the skin, and a very limited range of motion. Laboratory work-up was as follows: WBC count 9100/mm^3 with 75% polymorphonuclear cells and 17% lymphocytes; C-reactive protein (CRP) level 215 mg/L; erythrocyte sedimentation rate 47 mm/h, and a negative blood culture. The findings of a magnetic resonance imaging of the right ankle and foot with and without gadolinium were in keeping with the advanced infectious process of the ankle (Fig. 7.1). The patient was started on vancomycin and tazocin. On June 22, 2013, he underwent incision and drainage of deep right ankle abscesses. Tissue and pus were sent for Gram staining, aerobic and anaerobic bacterial cultures, acid-fast bacilli smear and culture, and *Mycobacterium tuberculosis* complex PCR, brucella culture, potassium hydroxide (KOH) smear and fungal culture, and 16S ribosomal RNA PCR and cytology. On July 2, the patient was discharged on levofloxacin, 750 mg/day and rifampin 600 mg daily. All the requested tests done at AUBMC were negative. In July 8, the 16S RNA PCR, which was referred to Bioscientia Reference Laboratories, Ingelheim, Germany, was positive and gene sequencing identified the organism as *U. urealyticum*.

Upon follow-up in clinic, the patient improved markedly with a decrease in the CRP level from 215 to 2.3 mg/L. He was switched to doxycycline, 100 mg twice a day to complete an 8-week course of antibiotics, after which he fully recovered.

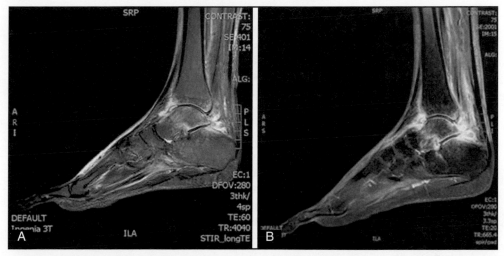

FIGURE 7.1 MRI of the right ankle and foot. (A) Sagittal short T1 inversion recovery (STIR) view shows large subcutaneous complex collection in the posteromedial aspect of the ankle extending to the Achilles tendon. There is ankle joint effusion with thickened enhancing joint capsule in keeping with septic arthritis; along with significant enhancing bone marrow edema in the posterior aspect of the calcaneus, in keeping with osteomyelitis. (B) Same view with STIR with gadolinium showing significant enhancement.

DISCUSSION

U. urealyticum belongs to the Mollicutes class of bacteria, which is also known as Mycoplasma. The organisms in this class are smaller than the traditional bacteria and lack a cell wall. Ureaplasma is known to have 14 serotypes, divided into two biovars: *Ureaplasma parvum* and *U. urealyticum*. Ureaplasmas are known to synthesize ATP through urea hydrolysis. These characteristics make them very sensitive to the environment. Hence, they require special growth medium supplemented with sterols, fatty acid, amino acids, and nucleic acid precursors.

U. urealyticum is transmitted sexually or vertically, *in utero* or perinatally.[1] It is part of the normal flora of the urogenital tract of the adult female where it is found in 40%– 80% females[2] and in the adult men, 25%– 40%.[3]

PATHOGENESIS

U. urealyticum is considered to have low virulence in general.[4] However, in some studies and many case reports, this organism has been associated with local infections[3,5,6] and/or systemic spread.[7]

For instance, *U. urealyticum* was found to be one of the etiologic factors of symptomatic nongonococcal urethritis (5%–10%) in men[3,5,6]; another association was found to be between *U. urealyticum* and chronic prostatitis.[8]

In addition, the presence of *U. urealyticum* has been linked to some sperm abnormality and altered morphology.[9–13] Other studies suggested that *U. urealyticum* might have a role in male infertility,[13,14] in preterm labor, and risk of miscarriage.[15,16]

Furthermore, it appears that *U. urealyticum* might cause more severe disease and systemic spread in special populations, especially newborns and patients with altered B cell function and antibody deficiencies such as hypogammaglobulinemia, and common variable immunodeficiency.[17,18] Other high risk diseases mentioned in the literature include: renal transplant,[19] lymphoma on chemotherapy in combination with rituximab,[20] systemic lupus erythematosus treated with rituximab,[21] and acute lymphoblastic leukemia[22]. The diseases seen in these high risk patients are mostly osteomyelitis[23,24] and septic arthritis[20,21,25] with rarely bacteremia[25] and one case of brain abscess.[26]

DIAGNOSIS

The diagnosis is often delayed[25] due to the limitations of culture, the gold standard for the diagnosis of *U. urealyticum;* it is further delayed when the clinical picture is not typically caused by Ureaplasma as in our case. Molecular-based techniques are more sensitive than culture[27]; they are capable of detecting even a small number of bacteria and might shorten the time to diagnosis. There are several reports in the literature of *U. urealyticum* infections diagnosed using molecular techniques.[28–30]

TREATMENT

Although not well standardized and poorly correlated with clinical outcomes, *in vitro* susceptibility testing shows that Ureaplasma species are susceptible to the tetracyclines (doxycycline) with very low resistance detected, approximately 5%.[31] They are also susceptible to clarithromycin, azithromycin, moxifloxacin, and ofloxacin, but not susceptible to clindamycin.

Patients with disease caused by Ureaplasma species should be treated. However, colonized patients do not require treatment.

CONCLUSION

When faced with negative standard cultures and PCRs for chlamydia and gonorrhea in sexually active patients with altered B cell function who present with septic arthritis or other deep-seated infections, clinicians should suspect *U. urealyticum* as a potential pathogen.

Molecular-based techniques such as the 16S ribosomal RNA-PCR provides a rapid technique for detection of fastidious and slowly growing bacteria, especially when the patient has been receiving antibiotic therapy for a long period of time. Even though it is not yet included in the current guidelines for the diagnosis of joint infections,[32] 16S ribosomal RNA-PCR (or molecular diagnostic methods) is useful in combination with routine microbiological tests to diagnose unusual infections in immunosuppressed patients.

QUESTIONS

1. What is the differential diagnosis of septic arthritis in a patient with high risk sexual activity?
2. What are the studies to be requested on the synovial fluid if the routine cultures are negative?
3. What are the risk factors that predispose *Ureaplasma urealyticum* septic arthritis?
4. What is the proper management of septic arthritis?
5. What type of infections can be caused by *Ureaplasma urealyticum,* as described in the literature?

REFERENCES

1. Sánchez PJ, Regan JA. Vertical transmission of *Ureaplasma urealyticum* from mothers to preterm infants. *Pediatr Infect Dis J.* 1990;9(6):398–401.
2. Waites KB, Katz B, Schelonka RL. Mycoplasmas and Ureaplasmas as neonatal pathogens. *Clin Microbiol Rev.* 2005;18(4):757–789.
3. Shahmanesh M, Moi H, Lassau F, Janier M, IUSTI/WHO. 2009 European guideline on the management of male non-gonococcal urethritis. *Int J STD AIDS.* 2009;20(7):458–464.
4. Waites KB, Schelonka RL, Xiao L, Grigsby PL, Novy MJ. Congenital and opportunistic infections: Ureaplasma species and *Mycoplasma hominis*. *Semin Fetal Neonatal Med.* 2009;14(4):190–199.
5. Shimada Y, Ito S, Mizutani K, et al. Bacterial loads of *Ureaplasma urealyticum* contribute to development of urethritis in men. *Int J STD AIDS.* 2014;25(4):294–298.
6. Povlsen K, Bjørnelius E, Lidbrink P, et al. Relationship of *Ureaplasma urealyticum* biovar 2 to nongonococcal urethritis. *Eur J Clin Microbiol Infect Dis.* 2002;21(2):97–101.
7. Larsen B, Hwang J. Mycoplasma, Ureaplasma, and adverse pregnancy outcomes: a fresh look. *Infect Dis Obstet Gynecol.* 2010;2010.
8. Radonifá A, Kovacevifá V, Markotifá A, et al. The clinical significance of *Ureaplasma urealyticum* in chronic prostatitis. *J Chemother.* 2009;21(4):465–466.
9. Zhang Q, Xiao Y, Zhuang W, et al. Effects of biovar I and biovar II of *Ureaplasma urealyticum* on sperm parameters, lipid peroxidation, and deoxyribonucleic acid damage in male infertility. *Urology.* 2014;84(1):87–92.
10. Potts JM, Sharma R, Pasqualotto F, Nelson D, Hall G, Agarwal A. Association of *Ureaplasma urealyticum* with abnormal reactive oxygen species levels and absence of leukocytospermia. *J Urol.* 2000;163(6):1775–1778.
11. Wang Y, Liang CL, Wu JQ, Xu C, Qin SX, Gao ES. Do *Ureaplasma urealyticum* infections in the genital tract affect semen quality? *Asian J Androl.* 2006;8(5):562–568.
12. Fraczek M, Szumala-Kakol A, Jedrzejczak P, Kamieniczna M, Kurpisz M. Bacteria trigger oxygen radical release and sperm lipid peroxidation in in vitro model of semen inflammation. *Fertil Steril.* 2007;88 (4 Suppl):S1076–S1085.
13. Zhang ZH, Zhang HG, Dong Y, Han RR, Dai RL, Liu RZ. *Ureaplasma urealyticum* in male infertility in Jilin Province, North-east China, and its relationship with sperm morphology. *J Int Med Res.* 2011;39(1):33–40.
14. Liu J, Wang Q, Ji X, et al. Prevalence of *Ureaplasma urealyticum, Mycoplasma hominis, Chlamydia trachomatis* infections, and semen quality in infertile and fertile men in China. *Urology.* 2014;83(4):795–799.
15. Padmini E, Uthra V. Role of *Ureaplasma urealyticum* in altering the endothelial metal concentration during preeclampsia. *Placenta.* 2012;33(4):304–311.
16. Padmini E, Uthra V, Lavanya S. HSP70 overexpression in response to *Ureaplasma urealyticum*-mediated oxidative stress in preeclamptic placenta. *Hypertens Pregnancy.* 2011;30(2):133–143.
17. Franz A, Webster AD, Furr PM, Taylor-Robinson D. Mycoplasmal arthritis in patients with primary immunoglobulin deficiency: clinical features and outcome in 18 patients. *Br J Rheumatol.* 1997;36(6):661–668.
18. Furr PM, Taylor-Robinson D, Webster AD. Mycoplasmas and Ureaplasmas in patients with hypogammaglobulinaemia and their role in arthritis: microbiological observations over twenty years. *Ann Rheum Dis.* 1994;53(3):183–187.
19. Cordtz J, Jensen JS. Disseminated *Ureaplasma urealyticum* infection in a hypo-gammaglobulinaemic renal transplant patient. *Scand J Infect Dis.* 2006;38(11-12):1114–1117.
20. Arber C, Buser A, Heim D, et al. Septic polyarthritis with *Ureaplasma urealyticum* in a patient with prolonged agammaglobulinemia and B-cell aplasia after allogeneic HSCT and rituximab pretreatment. *Bone Marrow Transplant.* 2007;40(6):597–598.
21. Goulenok TM, Bialek S, Gaudart S, Bébéar C, Fantin B. *Ureaplasma urealyticum* destructive septic arthritis in a patient with systemic lupus erythematosus after rituximab therapy. *Joint Bone Spine.* 2011;78(3):323–324.
22. Balsat M, Galicier L, Wargnier A, et al. Diagnosis of *Ureaplasma urealyticum* septic polyarthritis by PCR assay and electrospray ionization mass spectrometry in a patient with acute lymphoblastic leukemia. *J Clin Microbiol.* 2014;52(9):3456–3458.
23. Mohiuddin AA, Corren J, Harbeck RJ, Teague JL, Volz M, Gelfand EW. *Ureaplasma urealyticum* chronic osteomyelitis in a patient with hypogammaglobulinemia. *J Allergy Clin Immunol.* 1991;87(1 Pt 1):104–107.

24. Frangogiannis NG, Cate TR. Endocarditis and *Ureaplasma urealyticum* osteomyelitis in a hypogammaglobu-linemic patient. A case report and review of the literature. *J Infect.* 1998;37(2):181–184.
25. Asmar BI, Andresen J, Brown WJ. *Ureaplasma urealyticum* arthritis and bacteremia in agammaglobulinemia. *Pediatr Infect Dis J.* 1998;17(1):73–76.
26. Deetjen P, Maurer C, Rank A, Berlis A, Schubert S, Hoffmann R. Brain abscess caused by *Ureaplasma urea-lyticum* in an adult patient. *J Clin Microbiol.* 2014;52(2):695–698.
27. Waites KB, Xiao L, Paralanov V, Viscardi RM, Glass JI. Molecular methods for the detection of Mycoplasma and Ureaplasma infections in humans: a paper from the 2011 William Beaumont Hospital Symposium on molecular pathology. *J Mol Diagn.* 2012;14(5):437–450.
28. Vittecoq O, Schaeverbeke T, Favre S, et al. Molecular diagnosis of *Ureaplasma urealyticum* in an immunocom-petent patient with destructive reactive polyarthritis. *Arthritis Rheum.* 1997;40(11):2084–2089.
29. Schaeverbeke T, Renaudin H, Clerc M, et al. Systematic detection of mycoplasmas by culture and polymerase chain reaction (PCR) procedures in 209 synovial fluid samples. *Br J Rheumatol.* 1997;36(3):310–314.
30. Taylor-Robinson D, Gilroy CB, Horowitz S, Horowitz J. *Mycoplasma genitalium* in the joints of two patients with arthritis. *Eur J Clin Microbiol Infect Dis.* 1994;13(12):1066–1069.
31. Krausse R, Schubert S. In-vitro activities of tetracyclines, macrolides, fluoroquinolones and clindamycin against *Mycoplasma hominis* and *Ureaplasma ssp.* isolated in Germany over 20 years. *Clin Microbiol Infect.* 2010;16(11):1649–1655.
32. Baron EJ, Miller JM, Weinstein MP, et al. A guide to utilization of the microbiology laboratory for diagnosis of infectious diseases: 2013 recommendations by the Infectious Diseases Society of America (IDSA) and the American Society for Microbiology (ASM)(a). *Clin Infect Dis.* 2013;57(4):e22–e121.

Chapter 8

Campylobacter Prosthetic Valve Endocarditis

Manal Hamdan, Dina Mahmassani, and Nesrine Rizk

ABSTRACT

Prosthetic valve endocarditis is a destructive cardiac condition that can result in significant morbidity and mortality. It is the result of bacterial infection of the prosthetic device and could lead to valvular failure and valve replacement. *Campylobacter fetus* is rarely associated with infective endocarditis. Invasive disease with *C. fetus* is usually diagnosed by bacterial cultures and molecular techniques.

In this chapter, we describe a rare case of a prosthetic valve endocarditis due to *C. fetus*. The patient was a 36-year-old man who presented with acute onset of aphasia and right-sided weakness; those symptoms were preceded by 4 days of fever. The patient was suspected to have an ischemic stroke. He had no heart murmurs. A transesophageal echocardiogram showed two small masses noted on the ventricular surface of the prosthetic aortic valve annulus. Empiric antibiotic therapy was initiated for the treatment of a prosthetic valve endocarditis. The blood cultures showed *Campylobacter* species on the third day of admission. Bacterial 16S rDNA PCR testing on the aortic valve tissue revealed *C. fetus*. The antibiotic treatment regimen was adjusted according to the bacterial identification and antibiogram.

This chapter provides an overview of the rare published case reports of *Campylobacter* prosthetic valve endocarditis, including clinical manifestations, diagnosis, transmission, antibiotic therapy, duration of treatment, and outcome.

INTRODUCTION

Campylobacter fetus is an unusual cause of invasive human disease and particularly of prosthetic valve endocarditis with only a handful of cases reported in the literature.[1] We report a case of *C. fetus* prosthetic valve endocarditis in a patient with alcohol dependence and regular raw meat consumption. The presentation was complicated by neurologic events that prompted surgical intervention. There are currently no guidelines that dictate the management of prosthetic valve endocarditis, including the antibiotic choice and course of therapy. We will include a review of the prosthetic valve endocarditis cases reported in the literature and the management.

PATIENT CASE PRESENTATION

A 36-year-old man presented on June 8, 2015, at 1 a.m. to the Emergency Department with an acute onset of expressive aphasia associated with difficulty in swallowing, right-sided facial weakness, facial palsy, and right upper extremity weakness of 6-h duration. The symptoms were preceded by a 4-day history of high-grade fever and chills.

Three weeks prior to presentation, the patient reported consuming undercooked pork meat at a barbecue at home, and developing an acute diarrheal illness of 2-day duration. He did not receive antibiotics at the time. The patient had no recent dental work and no weight loss.

The patient's past medical history was significant for hypertension, G6PD deficiency, rheumatic heart disease, and a metallic aortic valve replacement (mechanical bileaflet aortic valve prosthesis) in 2007. He was maintained on anticoagulation and had a history of anaphylaxis to aspirin.

A year prior to presentation, in July 2014, the patient suffered from a similar febrile illness; he was diagnosed with brucellosis and treated with oral rifampin and doxycycline for 4 weeks. Later that year, our patient had two episodes of transient ischemic attacks with no permanent sequalae (August 2014: aphasia for 2 weeks, March 2015: aphasia for 4 weeks, right-sided weakness). Those episodes were attributed to inadequate anticoagulation secondary to poor compliance with medication intake.

The patient was married, lived with his wife and two young children in a rural area in the North of Lebanon. He owned a liquor store, ate raw and undercooked meat (pork and sheep). He was a heavy smoker and drank alcohol in excess, more than 15 beers per day. He also suffered from depression and attempted suicide in 2007.

On presentation, he had a temperature of 37.8°C, a blood pressure of 121/83 mm Hg, and a heart rate of 83 beats per minute. There was no skin rash or petechiae; he had no carotid bruit or cardiac murmurs. Poor dentition was noted on oral exam, and the neurologic exam was notable for an expressive aphasia, severe dysarthria, right peripheral facial palsy, and a weak right hand grip 4/5.

On laboratory studies, the white blood cell count was within normal range (7400/mm^3). C-reactive protein (CRP) level and erythrocyte sedimentation rate (ESR) were elevated at 33.1 mg/L and 46 mm/h, respectively. A computed tomography (CT) angiography of the head showed an acute left frontal infarct in Broca's area in addition to an old right frontal lacunar infarct. A transesophageal echocardiogram done on the same day showed two small (6–7 mm) masses noted on the ventricular surface of the prosthetic aortic valve annulus.

On the basis of these findings, a prosthetic valve endocarditis was suspected; three sets of blood were taken for culture (each consisting of one aerobic and one anaerobic bottle), and antibiotics were started. The antibiotic regimen included vancomycin, gentamicin, and ceftriaxone initially. The definite diagnosis of prosthetic valve endocarditis was established based on the modified Duke criteria for infective endocarditis, as the patient met one major criterion (evidence of endocardial involvement by an echocardiogram positive for vegetation) and four minor criteria (predisposing heart condition, i.e., prosthetic valve; fever; vascular phenomenon, i.e., major arterial emboli; and finally, microbiologic evidence with three positive blood cultures that did not meet Duke's major criteria).

On the third day of admission, the anaerobic blood culture bottles all grew Gram-negative rods (after 42, 22, and 51 h), later identified as *Campylobacter* species by Vitek 2-API. The Susc test showed R to cipro, and S to erythromycin (Clinical and Laboratory Standards Institute [CLSI] guidelines). PCR testing on the aortic valve tissue was performed at Bioscientia Reference Laboratories, Ingelheim, Germany. The sequencing of the amplified species-specific sections of the bacterial 16S rDNA by Light-Cycler revealed *C. fetus*.

The patient's fever resolved on the third day. There was a slight neurologic improvement and he underwent a dental evaluation. All blood cultures repeated negative at day 5. The patient underwent a Redo Aortic Valve Replacement (AVR) with size 25 Hancock porcine valve. We initiated imipenem and gentamicin intravenously.

Speech improved with therapy, and the patient was advised to continue speech therapy as well as physical therapy for right hand weakness after discharge.

DISCUSSION

We report a case of *C. fetus* prosthetic valve endocarditis complicated by septic emboli to the brain, and subsequent neurologic sequalae.

More than 15 different *Campylobacter* species have been identified. *C. fetus*, comprising 2 subspecies—*C. fetus* subspecies fetus (referred to as *C. fetus*) and *C. fetus* subspecies venerealis—can cause illness in humans as well as animals.[2] *C. fetus* subspecies fetus is an omnipresent pathogen, causing infections that mainly lead to abortion in cattle and sheep.

Some *C. fetus* infection case reports have described indirect transmission through raw milk,[3] insufficiently cooked chicken, beef or sheep meat or liver,[4] khat chewing,[5] inoculation via a peritoneal dialysis catheter,[6] and among slaughterhouse workers.[7]

Campylobacter species, including *C. fetus*, are unusual causes of endocarditis.

C. fetus is thought to be acquired through direct contact with infected hosts or via the ingestion of raw meat, as it was the case with this patient.[1,8]

Several other clinical syndromes related to *C. fetus* have been encountered, including bacteremia, infectious diarrhea, cholecystitis, peritonitis, septic arthritis, meningo-encephalitis, subdural empyema, lung abscesses, uterine infections, and cellulitis.[9]

The standard method for detecting *Campylobacter* species in clinical specimens is by laboratory culture, often by *Campylobacter* blood agar plates.[10] Given the fastidious nature of the organism, incubation of blood cultures is routinely extended to 2 weeks, when a systemic infection is suspected.

Growth is optimized in temperatures ranging between 37°C and 42°C.[10]

Campylobacter is a Gram-negative rod of comma or spiral shape (curved). Its motility is secondary to one or two polar flagellae. It is fastidious, slow growing, microaerophilic, nonspore forming, and does not ferment carbohydrates. Important biochemical reactions are nitrate reduction, H_2S production, catalase and oxidase activity, and growth in 1% glycine or bile.[11] Other methods for the direct detection of *Campylobacter* in clinical specimens, such as DNA probes and amplification by PCR, have been successful in research studies, and may be more sensitive than traditional cultures for the detection of and typing of these organisms.[12] It was first isolated from human infection by Vinzent.[13]

The pathogenesis of *C. fetus* has been well defined from all *Campylobacter* infections, although it is uncommon. Early studies identified a loosely-attached capsular envelope, surface (S)-layer protein from *C. fetus* that was later shown to render the organism's resistance to phagocytosis and complement-mediated killing. Moreover, the ability of the organism to switch surface-layer protein is believed to permit the organism's persistence in an immunologically hostile environment, especially in compromised hosts.[14]

In this case, we suspect that the infection was secondary to the ingestion of raw meat, with transintestinal migration of bacteria resulting in bacteremia and then ultimately prosthetic valve infection.

Several risk factors are related to *C. fetus* infection including aging, male sex (76%), implanted medical devices, immunocompromised state (diabetes mellitus, cancer, steroid therapy, HIV infection, liver diseases including cirrhosis, and alcohol abuse), but 26% of patients usually have no underlying disease.[15–17] In the literature, there are a few reports of infective endocarditis due to this microorganism, mainly among patients with valvular abnormalities or cardiomyopathy.

Only 30 cases of *C. fetus* endocarditis have been reported, predominantly among middle-aged men with an affected aortic valve.[18,19]

To our knowledge, only five previous cases of prosthetic valve endocarditis have been reported up to this date. There are no guidelines that dictate the antibiotic choice or course for the treatment of prosthetic valve endocarditis with *Campylobacter* species. The published cases are summarized in Table 8.1.

Three patients with bioprosthetic valves were treated with antibiotic combinations (including gentamicin) and valve replacement, and all three patients were cured.

In a fourth case, described by Peetermans et al.,[9] surgical repair was not done due to severe triple vessel coronary artery disease, and the patient died from complications related to severe infection.

In a case reported by Haruyama et al.,[1] the patient refused surgery and recovered after a prolonged course of combination antibiotic therapy with imipenem/cilastatin and gentamicin.

In the most recent reported case by Reid MJ et al.,[12] surgery was initially deferred but proved to be the definitive therapy after treatment failure with antibiotics alone.

According to the 2009 data of the French National Referral Centre for Campylobacter and Helicobacter, nearly 20% of *C. fetus* strains are resistant to ciprofloxacin and doxycycline and 10% are resistant to erythromycin.[21] Fluoroquinolones use was significantly associated with higher mortality of patients with *C. fetus* bacteremia.[15] Cefotaxime activity is poorer than that of the other beta-lactams. i.v. imipenem–aminoglycoside for weeks remains the recommended treatment for severe infections.[22] Imipenem resistance was reported only once.[23]

Our patient received i.v. imipenem and gentamicin for 4 weeks following the AVR. Bacteremia was cleared. The blood cultures taken 2 weeks after the surgery were negative and therefore, i.v. antibiotics were discontinued after a month and he did not suffer any complications (nephrotoxicity or ototoxicity). It was decided to deescalate to an oral macrolide, in this situation, azithromycin, for an additional 2 weeks.

He was still doing well 6 months after completing therapy.

QUESTIONS

1. What are common infections acquired from ingestion of raw meat?
2. What are the sources and transmission of Campylobacter pathogenic species?
3. What are the most common infections associated with Campylobacter?
4. What are the modified Duke criteria for endocarditis?
5. What are possible complications of endocarditis?

TABLE 8.1 Summary of Reported Cases of Prosthetic Valve Endocarditis Caused by *Campylobacter fetus*

Author	Age/sex	Comorbidities	Transmission	Operation, Valve Type	Postoperative Period	Antibiotics, Duration	Surgery	Outcome
Caramelli et al. (1988)[20]	48/F	Unknown	Unknown	MVR (bioprosthetic)	9 years	PCG + SM Then PCG + GM	Yes	Cured
Farrugia et al. (1994)[8]	76/F	Unknown	Unknown	AVR (bioprosthetic)	3 years	AMX + GM Then Cipro	Yes	Cured
Peetermans et al. (2000)[9]	61/M	Peptic ulcer disease	Unknown	AVR (mechanical)	26 years	EM + GM	No	Right atrium and ventricle abscess; Dead
Haruyama et al. (2011)[1]	65/F	Unknown	Raw meat Dental caries with toothache	Bentall procedure (bioprosthetic)	7 years	AMP + GM Then AMX Then IPM + GM	No	Cured
Reid et al. (2016)[12]	70/M	HTN Dyslipidemia	Steak tartare Dental cleaning	AVR (bioprosthetic)	4 years	MPM Then EPM	Yes	Cured
Case of this report (2016)	36/M	HTN G6PD deficiency Depression TIAs Alcoholic	Raw and undercooked meat (pork and sheep)	AVR (mechanical)	8 years	IPM + GM + CRT Then AZT	Yes	Cured

Notes: AMP, ampicillin; AMX, amoxicillin; AVR, aortic valve replacement; AZT, azithromycin; Cipro, ciprofloxacin; CRT, clarithromycin; EM, erythromycin; EPM, ertapenem; F, female; GM, gentamicin; IPM, imipenem; M, male; MPM, meropenem; MVR, mitral valve replacement; PCG, benzylpenicillin; SM, streptomycin.
Source: Modified with permission from Haruyama et al.[1] (Copyright 2011 by the Texas Heart Institute, Houston.)

REFERENCES

1. Haruyama A, Toyoda S, Kikuchi M, et al. *Campylobacter fetus* as cause of prosthetic valve endocarditis. *Tex Heart Inst J.* 2011;38(5):584–587.
2. Wagenaar JA, Bergen MA, Newell DG, Grogono-Thomas R, Duim B. Comparative study using amplified fragment length polymorphism fingerprinting, PCR genotyping, and phenotyping to differentiate *Campylobacter fetus* strains isolated from animals. *J Clin Microbiol* 2001;39:2283–2286.
3. Klein BS, Vergeront JM, Blaser MJ, et al. Campylobacter infection associated with raw milk. An outbreak of gastroenteritis due to *Campylobacter jejuni* and thermotolerant *Campylobacter fetus* subsp fetus. *JAMA.* 1986; 255:361–364.
4. Kramer JM, Frost JA, Bolton FJ, Wareing DR. Campylobacter contamination of raw meat and poultry at retail sale: identification of multiple types and comparison with isolates from human infection. *J Food Prot.* 2000;63:1654–1659.
5. Martínez-Balzano C, Kohlitz PJ, Chaudhary P, Hegazy H. *Campylobacter fetus* bacteremia in a young healthy adult transmitted by khat chewing. *J Infect* 2011;66:184–186.
6. Romero Gómez MP, García-Perea A, Ruiz Carrascoso G, Bajo MA, Mingorance J. *Campylobacter fetus* peritonitis and bacteremia in a patient undergoing continuous ambulatory peritoneal dialysis. *J Clin Microbiol.*2010;48:336–337.
7. Rennie RP, Strong D, Taylor DE, Salama SM, Davidson C, Tabor H. *Campylobacter fetus* diarrhea in a Hutterite colony: epidemiological observations and typing of the causative organism. *J Clin Microbiol.* 1994;32:721–724.
8. Farrugia DC1, Eykyn SJ, Smyth EG. *Campylobacter fetus* endocarditis: two case reports and review. *Clin Infect Dis.* 1994;18(3):443–446.
9. Peetermans WE, De Man F, Moerman P, van de Werf F. Fatal prosthetic valve endocarditis due to *Campylobacter fetus.* *J Infect* 2000;41(2):180–182.
10. M'Ikanatha NM, Dettinger LA, Perry A, et al. Culturing stool specimens for *Campylobacter spp.,* Pennsylvania, USA. *Emerg Infect Dis* 2012;18:484–487.
11. Schmidt U, Chmel H, Kaminski Z, et al. The clinical spectrum of *Campylobacter fetus* infections: report of five cases and review of the literature. *Q J Med.* 1980 Autumn;49(196):431–442.
12. Reid MJ, Shannon EM, Baxi SM, et al. Steak tartare endocarditis. *BMJ Case Rep.* 2016;2016. pii: bcr2015212928. doi: 10.1136/bcr-2015-212928.
13. McFaydean F; Stockman S. *Report of Departmental Committee.*1909.
14. Miki K1, Maekura R, Hiraga T, et al. Infective tricuspid valve endocarditis with pulmonary emboli caused by *Campylobacter fetus* after tooth extraction. *Intern Med.* 2005;44(10):1055–1059.
15. Pacanowski J, Lalande V, Lacombe K, et al. Campylobacter bacteremia: clinical features and factors associated with fatal outcome. *Clin Infect Dis.* 2008;47:790–796.
16. Gazaigne L, Legrand P, Renaud B, et al. *Campylobacter fetus* bloodstream infection: risk factors and clinical features. *Eur J Clin Microbiol Infect Dis.* 2008;27:185–189.
17. Suy F, Le Dû D, Roux AL, Hanachi M, Dinh A, Crémieux AC. Meningitis and endocarditis caused by *Campylobacter fetus* after raw-liver ingestion. *J Clin Microbiol.* 2013;51(9):3147-3150. doi: 10.1128/JCM.00631-13. Epub 2013 Jul 3.
18. Mahe I, Perdrix C, Maniere T, Holeman A, Diemer M, Bergmann JF. A case of *Campylobacter fetus* endocarditis of the tricuspid valve unaccompanied by fever. *Am J Med.* 2001;111(5):418.
19. Morrison VA, Lloyd BK, Chia JK, et al. Cardiovascular and bacteremic manifestations of *Campylobacter fetus* infection: case report and review. *Rev Infect Dis* 1990;12:387–392.
20. Caramelli B, Mansur AJ, Grinberg M, Mendes CM, Pileggi F. *Campylobacter fetus* endocarditis on a prosthetic heart valve. *South Med J.* 1988; 81(6):802–803.
21. King L, Lehours P, Mégraud F. *Bilan de la surveillance des infections à Campylobacter chez l'homme en France en 2009—synthèse.* Institut de Veille Sanitaire, Saint-Maurice, France. http://www.invs.sante.fr/publications/2010/plaquette_campylobacter/plaquette_campylobacter.pdf.
22. Tremblay C, Gaudreau C, Lorange M. Epidemiology and antimicrobial susceptibilities of 111 *Campylobacter fetus* subsp. fetus strains isolated in Québec, Canada, from 1983 to 2000. *J Clin Microbiol.* 2003;41:463–466.
23. Mosca A, Del Gaudio T, Miragliotta G. Imipenem-resistant *Campylobacter fetus* bloodstream infection. *J. Chemother.*2010; 22:142.

Chapter 9

Pandrug-Resistant *Acinetobacter baumannii* Infections: Case Series, Contributing Factors, Outcomes, and Available Treatment Options

Dania Abdallah, Habiba El-Mchad, and Rima Moghnieh

ABSTRACT

Extensively drug-resistant *Acinetobacter baumannii* (XDR-AB) has become a worldwide problem. At present, certain strains have become resistant to all available antibiotics, including polymyxins and glycylcyclines, which are generally considered to be antibiotics of the last resort; these strains are referred to as pandrug-resistant *Acinetobacter baumannii* (PDR-AB). We report a case series of seven subjects with PDR-AB infections first identified in our health care institution during 2015. All infected patients were elderly, above 60 years of age, and suffered from multiple comorbidities, high severity of illness scores, and low performance status. Reported infections caused by PDR-AB included ventilator-associated pneumonia, complicated intra-abdominal infection, and bacteremia alone and with lower respiratory tract infection. All patients were treated with a combination of potentially synergistic broad-spectrum antibiotics, specifically carbapenems, colistin, and tigecycline. However, the majority of patients had unfavorable clinical and microbiological outcomes resulting in death.

INTRODUCTION

Antibiotic-resistant bacterial infections emerged as a novel pandemic at the turn of the century, resulting in the so-called "antibiotic resistance crisis."[1-3] Strains with resistance to multiple antibiotics have been identified in major Gram-positive and Gram-negative species, and no antibiotic class has escaped this relentless phenomenon.[4,5] Magiorakos and colleagues suggested stratification of acquired resistance according to the antibiotic classes to which the bacteria remain susceptible, and their proposed definitions have been used widely both in the literature and in daily clinical practice.[6]

Within some nonfermenting Gram-negative bacteria, such as *Acinetobacter baumannii*, resistance has evolved to most or even all available antimicrobial options, except polymyxins (colistin) and glycylcyclines (tigecycline), resulting in extremely drug-resistant (XDR) phenotypes.[6] The extensive use of these last resort antibiotics in hospital settings is worrisome, and clinical reports of pandrug resistance have begun to appear, thus potentially creating conditions resemblant of the "preantibiotic era."[7-10]

A. baumannii has been increasingly associated with nosocomial epidemics world-wide.[11,12] Of particular concern are its environmental resilience, resulting in sustained outbreaks, as well as its inherent and acquired mechanisms of resistance to antibiotics.[13,14] We describe a series of hospitalized patients colonized or infected with *A. baumannii,* resistant to all available antibiotic classes at a tertiary care hospital. We analyzed the dynamics of the outbreak and clinical characteristics of the patients, including antibiotic history as a major risk factor for the acquisition of resistant *A. baumannii*. We also report patient microbiological and clinical outcomes and infection-related and 3-month (infection-independent) mortality.

METHODS

Setting and Patients

This is a retrospective chart review and a descriptive analysis of seven adult patients in whom PDR-AB was identified between October 2015 and January 2016 at Makassed General Hospital (MGH), a 150-bed university hospital located in Beirut, Lebanon. In addition to the general medicine and surgery wards, this center comprises a 13-bed critical care unit including a 4-bed open-bay intensive care unit (ICU) and 9 single cubicles. The nurse to patient ratio in the ICU is 2:1. Infection control measures and environmental hygiene were applied during the study period according to the Centers for Disease Control and Prevention (CDC) recommendations for controlling the spread of multidrug-resistant organisms in a health care setting.[15] However, until the emergence of PDR-AB, some of the mechanical ventilation equipment, including the endotracheal tubes, were disinfected and sterilized using cold-sterilization processes and were shared among all ventilated patients inside and outside the ICU, including within the isolation unit. Hand hygiene compliance rates were approximately 50% at the time of the PDR-AB outbreak. The hospital's Institutional Review Board approved this study and no patient consent was needed due to its retrospective nature.

Data Collected from Patients' Medical Records

(1) Patient demographics, clinical characteristics, and comorbidities prior to PDR-AB isolation
(2) Acute Physiology and Chronic Health Evaluation II (APACHE II) score at admission and at the time of PDR-AB identification and patient performance status, as indicated by dependence in mobility, feeding, and toileting
(3) Site of PDR-AB isolation and type of organ system involvement: ventilator-associated pneumonia (VAP), complicated skin and soft tissue infections, complicated intra-abdominal infections (cIAI), urinary tract infections, blood stream infections (BSI), bone and joint infections, and surgical site infections
(4) Broad-spectrum antibiotic history, including carbapenems, colistin, and tigecycline, and management of PDR-AB infection
(5) Length of stay (LOS) inside and outside the ICU prior to PDR-AB acquisition
(6) Clinical and microbiological outcomes of PDR-AB infection
(7) Infection-related mortality and 3-month mortality

XDR Empiric Therapy Regimens

Due to the epidemiology and predominance of XDR-AB as a nosocomial organism in our hospital, the empiric treatment for nosocomial pneumonia (including VAP) or septic shock is carbapenems (meropenem, 1 g i.v. every 8 h or imipenem, 500 mg i.v. every 6 h) combined with colistimethate sodium (4–6 million international units (MIU)/day with no loading dose until October 2015; subsequently, the dosage regimen was modified to a loading dose of 9 MIU followed by a maintenance dose of 9 MIU/day) *with or without tigecycline* (100 mg i.v. loading dose followed by a maintenance dose of 50 mg i.v. every 12 h).

Microbiological Studies and Breakpoints of Resistance

Bacterial identification was performed according to standard microbiological procedures. Antibiotic susceptibility testing was performed using the Kirby–Bauer disc diffusion Mueller–Hinton agar (Oxoid Ltd.) according to standard procedure. Culture plates were incubated at 37°C for 24 h. *Escherichia coli* American Type Culture Collection (ATCC) 25922 and *Pseudomonas aeruginosa* ATCC 27853 were used as quality control organisms for susceptibility testing according to Clinical and Laboratory Standards Institute (CLSI) recommendations.[16] CLSI breakpoints for the available systemic antibiotics against *A. baumannii* at MGH were employed in determining susceptibility. However, no interpretation data were available for tigecycline susceptibility against *A. baumannii* from CLSI[16] or the European Committee on Antimicrobial Susceptibility Testing (EUCAST)[17] regardless of the testing method. Therefore, we applied the clinical breakpoints suggested by Jones et al.[18] (susceptible (S) ≥ 16 mm, intermediate (I) 13–15 mm, and resistant (R) ≤ 12 mm). Neither CLSI[16] nor EUCAST[17] guidelines provided disc diffusion zone diameter breakpoints for colistin susceptibility against *A. baumannii*, and CLSI and EUCAST recommended that colistin testing should be interpreted according to minimal inhibitory concentration (MIC) breakpoints of S ≤ 2/R ≥ 4 mg/L and S ≤ 2/R > 2 mg/L, respectively. In our center, colistin susceptibility was also determined using the disc diffusion method with the following breakpoints: S ≥ 11 mm and R ≤ 8 mm.[19]

Definitions

(1) Outbreak: "the occurrence of more cases of disease than expected in a given area or among a specific group of people over a particular period of time"[20]

(2) Index case: "the patient in an outbreak who is first noticed by the health authorities, and who makes them aware that an outbreak might be emerging"[21]

(3) Colonization: "the recovery of the organism cultured from any clinical specimen with no clinical signs or symptoms of infection and no treatment initiated or changed by the treating clinician, or documented as colonization by the infectious disease specialist"[22]

(4) *Acinetobacter*-related infections were defined according to established criteria.[22,23] Infections were classified as hospital-acquired when onset occurred > 48 h after hospital admission and was not present or incubating at that time.[22] Documented infections were defined according to standardized definitions of the Unites States National Healthcare Safety Network/Center of Disease Control and Prevention (NHSN/CDC).[23]

(5) Extensive drug resistance in *A. baumannii*: "non-susceptibility to at least one agent in all but two or more antimicrobial categories" (i.e., susceptibility to only one or two categories).[6] In this study, XDR-AB isolates were susceptible only to tigecycline and colistin. They were resistant to all other categories, including carbapenems, cephalosporins, antipseudomonal penicillins, fluoroquinolones, aminoglycosides, and trimethoprim–sulfamethoxazole (TMP–SMX). Susceptibility to sulbactam was not tested because it is not available in Lebanon.

(6) Pandrug resistance in *A. baumannii*: non-susceptibility to all tested antibiotics at MGH, including cephalosporins, aztreonam, carbapenems, aminoglycosides, fluoroquinolones, TMP–SMX, colistin, and tigecycline.[6]

(7) Clinical outcome was defined as clinical success, clinical failure, or undetermined. Success was the presence of partial or complete improvement of signs/symptoms of infection and the absence of the necessity to use a new antibiotic for 72 h after treatment regimen discontinuation. Failure was persistence or worsening of the initial infection requiring a change in antibiotic therapy or infection-related death occurring more than 48 h after treatment regimen initiation. An undetermined outcome was defined by insufficient data, death not directly related to the initial infection or occurring within the first 48 h of treatment, or addition of an antibacterial agent for another infection.[24,25]

(8) Microbiological outcome was defined as success, failure, superinfection, or undetermined. Success was defined as eradication or conversion from the initial positive culture that warranted antibiotic therapy to a negative culture. Failure was the persistent identification of the same organism after initiating antibiotic treatment for 72 h or more. Superinfection was the development of a new infection after treatment initiation that necessitated an addition or a change in the antibiotic regimen. An undetermined outcome resulted when a specimen was not available for estimation of outcome.[24,25]

(9) Mortality: 3-month mortality was defined as death occurring within 3 months of hospital admission. Infection-related mortality was defined as death attributed to persistent infection.

(10) A day of therapy (DOT) was counted as any day in which the patient was prescribed an antibiotic.[26]

RESULTS

Patient Characteristics and Underlying Medical Conditions

Seven patients, comprising four males and three females, were identified to harbor PDR-AB between mid-November 2015, and the beginning of December 2015 (Table 9.1). They were mostly elderly, and five of the seven patients were above 60 years of age. All patients, except one, had comorbidities including cardiovascular diseases, diabetes, cerebrovascular accidents, and cancer. The patients had poor performance status on admission, and all were bedridden for more than 3 months, fed by nasogastric or gastrostomy tube and not independent in their toilet habits. APACHE II score at admission ranged between 11 and 25 with a median of 16. All patients, except one, were under mechanical ventilation. Prior to PDR-AB acquisition, the median LOS was 13 days in the ICU and 25 days in the hospital overall.

TABLE 9.1 Demographic and Clinical Features and Outcomes of the Studied Cases with Pandrug-Resistant *Acinetobacter baumannii*

Patient	Age/Gender	Comorbidities	APACHE II Score Upon Admission	Site of Isolation	Infection/Colonization	Treatment	Clinical Outcome	Microbiological Outcome	LOS in ICU before +PDR-AB (Days)	LOS in Hospital before +PDR-AB (Days)	Infection-related Mortality	3-Month Mortality
1	47/M	CVA, VP shunt	16	DTA	VAP	COL, IMP	Failure	Failure	-	15	Yes	Yes
2	65/M	CAD, CKD, diabetes	14	Urine	Colonization	COL, MEM, TYG	Undetermined	Failure	25	30	No	Yes
3	77/M	Afib, ARI, GI bleeding, seizures	19	DTA	Colonization	COL, MEM	Undetermined	Undetermined	5	6	No	No
4	72/F	Diabetes, CVA, HTN	11	DTA	VAP	COL, MEM	Success	Failure	23	25	No	Yes
5	64/F	Colorectal and uterine cancer, colostomy	15	Wound	cIAI	COL, MEM, TYG, RIF	Failure	Failure	-	22	Yes	Yes
6	74/M	HTN, CKD, renal cell carcinoma, spleenectomy	25	Nasopharynx	Colorization	-	Undetermined	Undetermined	20	30	No	Yes
7	56/F	No	23	Blood	BSI	COL, MEM	Failure	Undetermined	13	27	Yes	Yes

Note: Afib, atrial fibrillation; APACHE II, Acute Physiology and Chronic Health Evaluation II; ARI, acute renal injury; BSI, bloodstream infection; CAD, coronary artery disease; cIAI, complicated intra-abdominal infection; CKD, chronic kidney disease; DTA, deep tracheal aspirate; COL, colistimethate; CVA, cerebrovascular accident; F, female; HTN, hypertension; IMP, imipenem; GI, gastrointestinal; LOS, length of stay; M, male; MEM, meropenem; PDR-AB, pandrug-resistant *Acinetobacter baumannii*; RIF, rifampin; TYG, tigecycline; VAP, ventilazor-associated pneumonia; VP, ventriculoperitoneal shunt; (+), positive.
All cases were bedridden, fed by nasogastric tube and had urinary Foley catheters upon admission. All were mechanically ventilated prior to PDR-AB isolation except for patient 5. Patient 3 was discharged home.

Outbreak Description

The index PDR-AB case was identified in an internal medicine ward (IM-1) on November 14, 2015 (Patient 1). This patient had previously acquired XDR-AB during the same admission and on the same floor on November 7, 2015 (Fig. 9.1). He was treated with

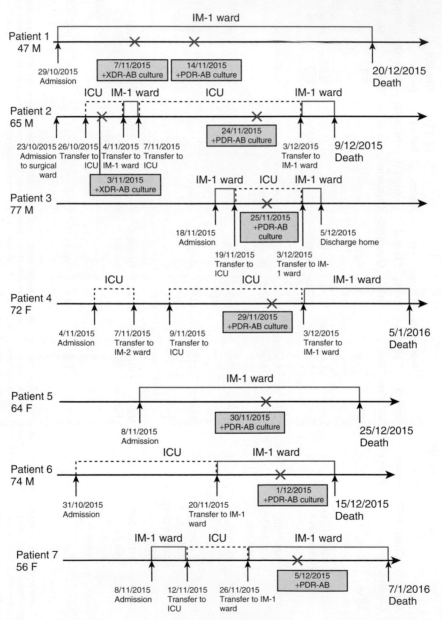

FIGURE 9.1   Timeline for each case showing transfer between wards and the date of pandrug-resistant *Acinetobacter baumanni* acquisition during the whole hospital stay.

(F, female; ICU, intensive care unit; IM, internal medicine; M, male; PDR-AB, pandrug-resistant *Acinetobacter baumannii;* XDR-AB, extensively drug-resistant *Acinetobacter baumannii;* (+), positive.)

Note: The internal medicine wards (IM-1 and IM-2) and the surgical ward are located each on a separate floor.

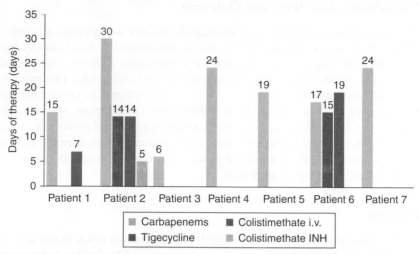

FIGURE 9.2 Days of therapy for carbapenems, tigecycline, and colistimethate sodium administered prior to the isolation of pandrug-resistant *Acinetobacter baumannii* in each of the seven cases.
Note: INH, inhaled; i.v., intravenous.

carbapenems for 7 days prior to XDR-AB isolation (Fig. 9.2). Ten days later, on November 24, 2015, the index case in the ICU (Patient 2) was identified; this patient was a carrier of XDR-AB and previously treated with carbapenems for 7 days and inhaled colistin for 5 days. During his hospital stay, Patient 2 was simultaneously present in IM-1 with Patient 1 between November 4 and November 7, 2015. Patients 2, 3, and 4 subsequently were admitted to the ICU within an average of 4 days apart. The ICU stays of these four patients overlapped, and all, except Patient 4, were admitted to IM-1 for a few days prior to PDR-AB isolation. On November 30, 2015, PDR-AB was identified in Patient 5 while admitted in the IM-1 ward; however, this patient had not been found to be previously colonized with XDR-AB and was not transferred from the ICU. Yet, this patient was present on the same floor with index Patient 1 for approximately 22 days prior to PDR-AB acquisition. On December 1 and 5, 2015, PDR-AB was identified in Patients 6 and 7, respectively, while admitted to IM-1 after being transferred from the ICU.

The outbreak was interrupted by environmental disinfection including bleach wiping (a 1:10 dilution of 5.25% sodium hypochlorite and water) followed by fumigation with 35% vaporized hydrogen peroxide achieving a room concentration of 320 ppm during 1-h contact time and another hour for aeration with ward closure, cessation of cold sterilization of single-use items, and 100% adherence to disposing single-use items according to manufacturers' instructions.

Antibiotic History

All patients received carbapenems prior to PDR-AB acquisition (Fig. 9.2). Carbapenem DOT during the 3 months prior to acquisition ranged from 6 to 30 days with a median of 19 days. Patients 1, 2, and 6 received i.v. colistin for 7, 14, and 19 days prior to PDR-AB isolation, respectively. Patient 2 also received inhaled colistin for 5 days before acquiring PDR-AB. Tigecycline was initiated in Patients 2 and 6 for 14 and 15 days, respectively, prior to PDR-AB emergence.

PDR-AB Isolation, Infection, and Outcome

Of the seven cases, three (Patients 2, 3, and 6) did not show any sign of infection, yet revealed urine, deep tracheal aspirate (DTA), and nasopharyngeal colonization, respectively (Table 9.1) The remaining four patients developed infections: Patients 1 and 4 had VAP; Patient 2 had cIAI postabdominal surgery; and Patient 7 had bacteremia. The treatment team initiated or continued antibiotic therapy in all cases as an attempt to control the outbreak. PDR-AB treatment was a combination of carbapenems (meropenem or imipenem) plus colistin with or without tigecycline or rifampin. Follow-up bacterial cultures were available in four patients who showed treatment failure. Clinical success was achieved in one of the four infected patients, and infection-related mortality occurred in three patients. Six patients died within 3 months of hospital admission.

DISCUSSION

This case series represents a PDR-AB outbreak involving seven cases in the ICU and in a general medicine ward of our health care facility between mid-November and the beginning of December 2015. Four of the seven patients developed PDR-AB infection.

    Antibiotic-resistant *Acinetobacter* infections have become a major cause of mortality among critically ill patients.[11] In the past, *Acinetobacter* was considered an organism of low virulence, predominately causing infections among immunocompromised hosts.[27] However, more recent data have shown that this species may exhibit substantial virulence, and, given the paucity of novel antibiotics, *Acinetobacter* infection is now recognized as a serious public health concern.[28]

    In one epidemiological study conducted by our hospital ICU in 2004, *Acinetobacter* represented 18.9% of the total isolated species, of which 20% were XDR.[29] In 2014, 90% of *Acinetobacter* species were carbapenem-resistant and 13% were resistant to tigecycline; however, no colistin resistance has been identified so far (unpublished hospital data). In a recent compilation of bacteriology data from 16 Lebanese hospitals between 2011 and 2013, XDR-AB represented 82% of the total *Acinetobacter* isolates, none of which were PDR.[30]

    On the basis of new recommendations for colistin dosing, we consider that patients with XDR-AB may be underdosed in our facility. Underdosage and prolonged exposure to colistin might have contributed to the emergence of colistin resistance. Markou et al.[31] assessed steady-state serum concentrations of colistin after intravenous administration of colistin methanesulfonate (CMS) in critically ill patients with stable kidney function. Even at steady state (at least 2 days after starting therapy), the reported plasma concentration was low despite a creatinine clearance >46 mL/min and administration of 2.8 MIU CMS intravenously every 8 or 12 h (corresponding to ~270 mg colistin base activity per day).[31] Markou et al.[31] concluded that maximum concentrations of colistin were probably not sufficient to ensure optimal maximum concentration (C_{max})/MIC ratios for *Acinetobacter* sensitive to colistin (MIC $\leq$ 2 mg/L). Similarly, cases in our study received the same dosage regimen; however, we hypothesize that at steady state, the plasma concentrations of formed colistin were below MIC breakpoints.

    Of major concern, the emergence of colistin-resistant *Acinetobacter* phenotypes has been found to be predominantly due to colistin heteroresistance, which is the presence of resistant subpopulations within an isolate that overall is considered to be susceptible based upon its MIC ($\leq$2 mg/L), previously described by Li et al.[32] The presence of these heteroresistant subpopulations suggests that colistin would best be used as part of a highly active combination (e.g., with rifampin), especially when treating an infection caused by an organism with an MIC $\geq$ 0.5 mg/L.[32]

Combination regimens used in the treatment of our patients comprised antibiotics; XDR-AB is nonsusceptible. Despite the fact that these antibiotics may be beneficial in treating concomitant infections caused by other susceptible organisms, they do not usually achieve plasma concentrations sufficient to eradicate XDR-AB, thus leading to colistin resistance. Several studies have assessed in vitro synergy testing of different antimicrobials against *Acinetobacter* by using time-kill and checkerboard assays.[33] The results of these studies have been inconsistent; therefore, no consensus has yet been reached regarding the best combination to be used.[33] Thus, we conclude that each health care facility should do its own synergy testing to determine the most suitable antimicrobial combination to use against its endemic strains.

In addition to its inherent and acquired mechanisms of resistance to antibiotics, PDR-AB transfer among patients due to cross-contamination via health care workers' hands, equipment, or the hospital environment is another key factor in the development of colonization or even infection.[13] In our series, the index case was identified while admitted in the IM-1 ward. After 10 days, PDR-AB acquisition was identified in the ICU and later on again in the same medical ward.

Another equally important factor in acquiring PDR-AB was that all our cases received carbapenems for prolonged periods of time (DOT, range: 6–30 days, median: 19 days), and the use of carbapenems was more consistent than the use of either colistin or tigecycline. In a recently published Lebanese study, carbapenem use was found to be a major risk factor for XDR-AB acquisition in the ICU by multivariate analysis.[34] Likewise, one study found that fluoroquinolones played a similar role,[35] and another study identified prior use of colistin as the only risk factor associated with emergence of colistin-resistant *Acinetobacter* phenotypes (odds ratio = 7.78, *p*-value < 0.002).[36] In another recent case series including 20 patients with PDR-AB, 19 of these patients had received intravenous and/or inhaled CMS for the treatment of carbapenem-resistant, colistin-susceptible *Acinetobacter* infection prior to identification of colistin-resistant isolates.[8]

Within all included patients, the basic performance status was poor, and total dependence on caregivers was identified. This critically ill category of patients may be subject to recurrent infections because of their level of debilitation, continuous exposure to invasive devices including central venous catheters, gastrostomy tubes, urinary catheters, and mechanical ventilation, and high risk of developing pressure ulcers and aspiration. Accordingly, they are also more likely to receive multiple courses of antibiotics. When these patients are colonized with XDR Gram-negative bacteria, the treatment choices become limited and repeating the same antibiotic course becomes unavoidable, which may lead to in vivo emergence of further resistance. Within 3 months of PDR-AB acquisition and within at least 30 days following admission, six of the seven patients died; the cause of death was infection-related in three. Falagas et al.[7] reported a series of 28 patients infected with pandrug-resistant Gram-negative organisms. Two of the patients in their study were infected with PDR-AB: one with central nervous system infection and the other with pneumonia. While both patients were aged less than 30 years, they had negative outcomes, likely due to major trauma.[7] Similarly, in another case series, the most common infection was VAP and the 30 days all-cause mortality rate reached 30%.[8] In comparison, our cases were much older (all older than 60 years) with multiple comorbidities and low performance status on admission, leading to a higher mortality rate. This observation opens the door to important research questions about the life expectancy of this category of patients after hospital admission and about the benefit of using last resort antimicrobials given their debilitation and cognitive status.

STUDY LIMITATIONS

One of the limitations of this study is that susceptibility to colistin and tigecycline in our center was determined using the disc diffusion method. Both CLSI[16] and EUCAST[17] guidelines recommend MIC determination for these two drugs with a breakpoint of 2 mg/L for colistin and an undetermined breakpoint for tigecycline. Disc diameter breakpoints have not yet been established in international guidelines.[16,17] Another drawback was that periodic screening cultures were not taken, and most of the cultures were diagnostic and taken when needed. However, this case series describes an outbreak caused by a highly virulent pandrug-resistant organism that is currently a worldwide public health concern. It is also a perfect example of the intertwining role of infection control and antimicrobial stewardship.

CONCLUSIONS

PDR-AB, as shown in this series, occurs mostly in patients with low performance status and subject to high mortality that is not necessarily infection related. Underdosing and prolonged exposure to last resort antimicrobials such as colistin and tigecycline may have caused the emergence of this pan resistance. Repeated courses of antimicrobials are a frequent component of clinical care for this critically ill category of patients who are prone to recurrent infections. Antimicrobial-dosing regimens should be designed according to pharmacokinetic and pharmacodynamic profiles, for example, higher dose and/or longer duration of i.v. infusions with high C_{max} or C_{max}/MIC values. Combination therapy is usually recommended and should be guided by in vitro synergy assays. Finally, effort should be made to eliminate risk factors for infection through rigorous infection control measures and judicious antibiotic use.

CONFLICT OF INTEREST STATEMENT

None declared.

FUNDING SOURCES

None.

QUESTIONS

1. What is the role of i.v. colistin underdosing and colistin heteroresistance in the emergence of PDR-AB strains?
2. Why is in vitro synergy testing of antibiotic combinations important?
3. How does the hospital environment favor PDR-AB transmission?
4. Do other factors play a role in PDR-AB emergence?
5. Who are the patients with the worst treatment outcomes?

REFERENCES

1. Rossolini GM, Arena F, Pecile P, Pollini S. Update on the antibiotic resistance crisis. *Curr Opin Pharmacol.* 2014, 18:56–60.
2. CDC. *Transatlantic Taskforce on Antimicrobial Resistance.* 2014.
3. WHO (World Health Organization). *Antimicrobial Resistance: Global Report on Surveillance.* 2014. http://apps.who.int/iris/bitstream/10665/112642/1/9789241564748_eng.pdf.
4. Willems RJL, Hanage WP, Bessen DE, Feil EJ. Population biology of Gram-positive pathogens: high-risk clones for dissemination of antibiotic resistance. *FEMS Microbiol Rev* 2011, 35:872–900.
5. Woodford N, Turton JF, Livermore DM. Multiresistant Gram-negative bacteria: the role of high-risk clones in the dissemination of antibiotic resistance. *FEMS Microbiol Rev* 2011, 35:736–755.
6. Magiorakos A-P, Srinivasan A, Carey RB, et al. Multidrug-resistant, extensively drug-resistant and pandrug-resistant bacteria: an international expert proposal for interim standard definitions for acquired resistance. *Clin Microbiol Infect* 2012, 18:268–281.
7. Falagas ME, Rafailidi PI, Matthaiou DK, Virtzili S, Nikita D, Michalopoulos A. Pandrug-resistant *Klebsiella pneumoniae*, *Pseudomonas aeruginosa* and *Acinetobacter baumannii* infections: characteristics and outcome in a series of 28 patients. *Int J Antimicrob Agents* 2008; 32(5): 450–454.
8. Qureshi ZA, Hittle LE, O'Hara JA, et al. Colistin-resistant *Acinetobacter baumannii*: beyond carbapenem resistance. *Clin Infect Dis.* 2015, civ048.
9. Apisarnthanarak A, Pinitchai U, Thongphubeth K, Yuekyen C, Warren DK, Fraser VJ. A multifaceted intervention to reduce pandrug-resistant *Acinetobacter baumannii* colonization and infection in 3 intensive care units in a Thai tertiary care center: a 3-year study. *Clin Infect Dis* 2008; 47(6): 760–767.
10. Jaidane N, Chaouech C, Messaoudi A, Boujaafar N, & Bouallegue O. Colistin-resistant *Acinetobacter baumannii*: a case report and literature review. *Rev Med Microb* 2015, 26(2), 78–83.
11. Falagas ME, Karveli EA, Siempos II, Vardakas KZ. Acinetobacter infections: a growing threat for critically ill patients. *Epidemiol Infect* 2008; 136: 1009–1019.
12. Perez F, Hujer AM, Hujer KM, Decker BK, Rather RN, Bonomo RA. Global challenge of multidrug resistant *Acinetobacter baumannii*. *Antimicrob Agents Chemother* 2007; 51: 3471–3484.
13. Villalón P, Valdezate S, Cabezas T, et al. Endemic and epidemic *Acinetobacter baumannii* clones: a twelve-year study in a tertiary care hospital. *BMC Microbiol* 2015;15:47.
14. Villegas MV, Hartstein AI. *Acinetobacter* outbreaks, 1977–2000. *Infect Control Hosp Epidemiol* 2003;24:284–295.
15. Rutala WA, Weber DJ; Healthcare Infection Control Practices Advisory Committee. Guideline for disinfection and sterilization in healthcare facilities. http://www.cdc.gov/hicpac/pubs.html; 2008. Accessed 24.11.16.
16. Clinical and Laboratory Standards Institute. *Performance Standards for Antimicrobial Susceptibility Testing; Twenty-Second Informational Supplement.* Clinical and Laboratory Standards Institute, 950 West Valley Road, Suite 2500, Wayne, Pennsylvania 19087 USA, 2012. CLSI document M100-S22 (ISBN 1-56238-785-5 [Print]; ISBN 1-56238-786-3 [Electronic]).
17. The European Committee on Antimicrobial Susceptibility Testing. Breakpoint Tables for Interpretation of MICs and Zone Diameters. Version 6.0. 2016. http://www.eucast.org.
18. Jones RN, Ferraro MJ, Reller LB, et al. Multicenter studies of tigecycline disk diffusion susceptibility results for Acinetobacter spp. *J Clin Microbiol* 2007; 45(1): 227–230.
19. Sınırtaş M, Akalın H, Gedikoğlu S. Investigation of colistin sensitivity via three different methods in *Acinetobacter baumannii* isolates with multiple antibiotic resistance. *Int J Infect Dis.* 2009;13(5):e217–e220.
20. Last JM. *A Dictionary of Epidemiology*, 4th ed. New York: Oxford U Press, 2001:129.
21. Johan Giesecke. Primary and index cases. *The Lancet* 2014; 384(9959): 2024
22. Garner JS, Jarvis WR, Emori TG, Horan TC, Hughes JM. CDC definitions for nosocomial infections. *Am J Infect Control* 1988;16:128–140.
23. Centers for Disease Control and Prevention. 2016 National Healthcare Safety Network (NHSN) Patient Safety Component manual. https://www.cdc.gov/nhsn/pdfs/pscmanual/pcsmanual_current.pdf; 2016. Accessed 24.11.16.
24. Montravers P, Dupont H, Bedos JP, et al. Tigecycline use in critically ill patients: a multicentre prospective observational study in the intensive care setting. *Intensive Care Med.* 2014; 40(7): 988–997.

25. Kuo SC, Wang FD, Fung CP, et al. Clinical experience with tigecycline as treatment for serious infections in elderly and critically ill patients. *J Microbiol, Immunol Infect.* 2011; 44(1):45–51.

26. Rhodes NJ, Wagner JL, Gilbert EM, Crew PE, Davis SL and Scheet MH. Days of therapy and antimicrobial days: similarities and differences between consumption metrics. *Infect Control Hosp Epidemiol* 2016;37(8): 971–973 doi:10.1017/ice.2016.109

27. Joly-Guillou ML. Clinical impact and pathogenicity of *Acinetobacter. Clin Microbiol Infect* 2005; 11(11): 868–873.

28. Gordon NC, Wareham DW. Multidrug-resistant *Acinetobacter baumannii*: mechanisms of virulence and resistance. *Int J Antimicrob Agents* 2010;35(3):219–226.

29. Abu Daher J, Shaar T, Lababidi H. Microorganisms profile and antimicrobial susceptibility in the intensive care unit: the emergence of a resistant pathogen–*Acinetobacter baumanii. Chest.* 2006;130 (4_meetingabstracts):217S. Doi:10.1378/chest.130.4_meetingabstracts.217S-a

30. Chamoun K, Farah M, Araj G, et al. Surveillance of antimicrobial resistance in Lebanese hospitals: retrospective nationwide compiled data. *Int J Infect Dis.* 2016;46:64–70.

31. Markou N, Markantonis SL, Dimitrakis E, et al. Colistin serum concentrations after intravenous administration in critically ill patients with serious multidrug-resistant, gram-negative bacilli infections: a prospective, open-label, uncontrolled study. *Clin Ther* 2008;30(1):143–151.

32. Li J, Rayner CR, Nation RL et al. Heteroresistance to colistin in multidrug-resistant *Acinetobacter baumannii. Antimicrob Agents Chemother* 2006; 50:2946–2950.

33. Gabriel A March, Miguel A Bratos. A meta-analysis of in vitro antibiotic synergy against *Acinetobacter baumannii. J Microbiol Methods* 2015; 119: 31–36.

34. Moghnieh R, Siblani L, Ghadban D, et al. Extensive drug-resistant *Acinetobacter baumanii* in a Lebanese Intensive Care Unit: risk factors for acquisition and determination of a colonisation score. *J Hosp Infect* 2016; 92(1):47–53.

35. Inchai J, Liwsrisakun C, Theerakittikul T, Chaiwarith R, Khositsakulchai W, Pothirat C. Risk factors of multi-drug-resistant, extensively drug-resistant and pandrug-resistant *Acinetobacter baumannii* ventilator-associated pneumonia in a Medical Intensive Care Unit of University Hospital in Thailand. *J Infect Chemother* 2015; 21(8):570–574.

36. Matthaiou DK, Michalopoulos A, Rafailidis PI, et al. Risk factors associated with the isolation of colistin-resistant gram-negative bacteria: a matched case-control study. *Crit Care Med* 2008;36:807–811.

Chapter 10

Candida parapsilosis Endocarditis on a Damaged Native Valve: A Case Report and Review of Management Options

Aia Assaf-Casals, Salim Musallam, Rouba Shaker, Zeinab El Zein,
Mohammad Abutaqa, Mariam Arabi, Issam Rassi, Fadi Bitar,
Ghassan Dbaibo, and Rima Hanna-Wakim

ABSTRACT

Candida is the most important cause of fungal infection in health care settings, affecting mainly immunocompromised patients, patients with critical illness, prematurity, or complex chronic conditions. It is now reported as the fourth most common cause of health care–associated bloodstream infections in children. One species, *Candida parapsilosis*, has emerged as a major human pathogen over the past two decades, and has become one of the leading causes of invasive candidiasis.

Candida endocarditis is a relatively new syndrome and is often a complication of medical and surgical advances. Despite aggressive combined medical and surgical interventions, mortality rates from fungal endocarditis are unacceptably high.

We report the case of a 10-month-old-female infant with cleft palate and atrioventricular (AV) canal malformation who developed persistent *C. parapsilosis* fungemia for 22 days despite appropriate antifungal therapy. During her hospital stay, the patient later developed 6 × 3 mm vegetation over the mitral valve. She underwent open heart surgery for removal of the vegetation 9 weeks into antifungal therapy. Culture of the vegetation grew *C. parapsilosis*. She received amphotericin B and flucytosine for a total of 4 months and was discharged home on oral fluconazole as suppressive therapy. Unfortunately, the patient passed away 1 week after discharge from sudden cardiac arrest.

Candida endocarditis has high mortality and relapse rates even with appropriate antifungal treatment. There is a lack of consensus on the appropriate management of these cases due to lack of prospective trials. Prolonged therapy with a combination of antifungals followed by suppressive therapy and surgical intervention, when possible, seems to be the most appropriate approach.

INTRODUCTION

Invasive candida infections are associated with significant morbidity and mortality, particularly in the hospital setting.[1–4] Candida is reported to be the fourth most common cause of bloodstream infections (BSI) worldwide but represents the second most common cause of central venous line associated infections.[4–6] Previously, *Candida albicans* was undoubtedly the most commonly isolated species but recently, nonalbicans species are increasingly being isolated.[1,6,7] One species, *Candida parapsilosis*, has emerged as a major human pathogen with an important role in nosocomial BSI over the past decade.[6,8–12]

Although relatively rare, fungal endocarditis carries serious complications with high morbidity and mortality.[13–15] *C. parapsilosis* is the second most common causative species after *C. albicans*.[16–18] Usually, prosthetic valves are involved and only rare reports of native valve candida endocarditis have been reported.[15,17–22] Even with early aggressive medical and surgical treatment, mortality remains high.[15]

CASE REPORT

History and Presenting Symptoms

We report a case of a 10-month-old-female infant with cleft palate on nasoduodenal feeding, AV canal malformation repaired 5 months earlier, severe gastro-esophageal reflux disease, chronic lung disease, neurodevelopmental delay, and frequent episodes of supraventricular tachycardia, who was admitted to our intensive care unit for the management of arrhythmia in April 2015. The patient had a history of recurrent admissions for similar complaints in addition to multiple infections. She had a right internal jugular Broviac® line inserted at the age of 5 months because of difficult peripheral intravenous access.

Examination

The patient was febrile and pale with mild respiratory distress. There was no erythema at the level of insertion of the Broviac® line. On auscultation, she had grade III/i.v. systolic ejection murmur with diffuse rhonchi.

Investigation

Central and peripheral blood cultures initially grew *Enterococcus faecalis*. Three days later, central and peripheral blood cultures grew *Candida spp.* that was later identified as *C. parapsilosis* sensitive to fluconazole (minimum inhibitory concentration MIC ≤ 1 mcg/mL), voriconazole (MIC ≤ 0.12 mcg/mL), caspofungin (MIC = 0.5 mcg/mL), and amphotericin B (MIC =1 mcg/mL). Echocardiography was done to rule out endocarditis and it was negative for any evidence of vegetation (Fig. 10.1A).

Diagnosis

C. parapsilosis endocarditis.

Management

The patient was started on appropriate antibiotics once blood cultures grew *E. faecalis*. Three days later, blood cultures had cleared from *E. faecalis* but grew *Candida spp.* The central line was urgently removed and she was started on liposomal amphotericin B. Daily blood cultures continued to grow *C. parapsilosis*, so flucytosine was added to amphotericin B around 2 weeks after the first positive culture. Follow-up echocardiography showed an echogenic focus over the anterior leaflet of the left AV valve, consistent with vegetation (Fig. 10.1B). Candidemia cleared 22 days after initiating antifungal therapy. Extensive

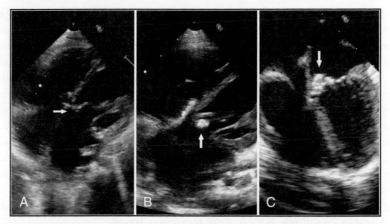

FIGURE 10.1   Echocardiography: (A) transthoracic echocardiography, four chamber view shows clean anterior leaflet of the left AV valve (arrow) with no evidence of vegetation; (B) transthoracic echocardiography, four chamber view shows an echogenic lesion over the atrial surface of the anterior leaflet of the left AV valve (arrow) consistent of vegetation; (C) intraoperative transesophageal echocardiography, four chamber view shows a larger vegetation (arrow), mobile, measuring 6 × 3 mm in dimension causing moderate to severe left atrioventricular valve insufficiency.

workup for a deep-seated fungal infection including dilated fundoscopy, CTs of the chest, abdomen, pelvis, and brain were nonrevealing. Serial echocardiographic studies showed an increase in the size of the vegetation up to 6 × 3 mm despite medical therapy, and it became mobile (Fig. 10.1C). Several multidisciplinary discussions were done and she underwent open heart surgery for removal of the vegetation 9 weeks into antifungal therapy. Culture of the resected vegetation grew *C. parapsilosis*. She gradually improved clinically. She received amphotericin B and flucytosine for a total of 4 months and was discharged home on oral fluconazole as suppressive therapy. Unfortunately, the patient passed away 1 week after discharge.

DISCUSSION

Candida has become an increasingly common cause of nosocomial infections with significant morbidity and mortality.[1–4] Risk factors for invasive candidemia include immunocompromised states, prematurity, critical illnesses, complex chronic conditions, prolonged antibiotic use, and presence of central venous catheters (CVCs).[23–25] CVC-associated BSI due to *Candida spp.* come only second to coagulase-negative *Staphylococcus* organisms.[12,23] There has been increased incidence of nonalbicans *Candida spp.* as an important cause of infections in health care settings compared to the relatively steady incidence of *C. albicans*.[6,23,26] In the past two decades, *C. parapsilosis* has emerged as one of the major pathogens in CVC-associated BSI infection owing to their characteristic adherence to prosthetic material by forming biofilms.[8,23,27] *C. parapsilosis* is frequently isolated from the subungual space and this emphasizes the importance of proper hand hygiene as a prevention strategy against hospital outbreaks.[8,27] Our patient had a 5-month-old central line with a history of multiple admissions that had required repeated handling of the central line by health care workers and thus increasing the risk of acquiring *C. parapsilosis*. Persistent candidemia observed in our patient has been reported in several patients mostly with debilitating conditions and resistant species.[28,29] One study reported the isolation of *C. parapsilosis* as a significant risk factor for persistent candidemia.[30] The presence of complex congenital and chronic diseases in our patient likely contributed to the persistent candidemia despite CVC removal and appropriate therapy. However, the most likely reason is probably the endocarditis, which probably was initiated as a result of the CVC infection and which evaded initial detection on repeated echocardiograms only to be firmly diagnosed 18 days into candidemia when a new AV valve vegetation was detected. The fact that the patient's left AV valve was repaired earlier by reinforcing sutures in the anterior leaflet is likely a significant predisposing factor for developing endocarditis. Another risk factor is the residual left AV valve regurgitation, secondary to the nature of the disease even prior to surgery since both the left and right AV valves were initially fused and abnormal. Also, the prolonged candidemia would expectedly increase the risk of renal, ophthalmic, and other deep-seated infections, but no other focus was found.

Fungal endocarditis is a rare and relatively new syndrome accounting for only 1.3–6% of infective endocarditis; nevertheless, it is associated with a high mortality rate reaching 50% even with appropriate treatment.[16,18,21,22,31,32] *C. albicans* is the most common cause followed by *C. parapsilosis* as observed in our case.[18] It is mostly isolated from prosthetic aortic and mitral valves, but few reports of native valve infection with *C. parapsilosis* have been published.[8,14–21,31,33] The most important risk factor for *C. parapsilosis* endocarditis reported is intravenous drug use, central line presence for long periods, and valvular disease.[8,18] A case series among pediatric patients with congenital heart disease (CHD) concluded that CHD is a risk factor for candidemia and consequently endocarditis. *C. parapsilosis* was the most commonly isolated organism in this specific population.[3]

Candida endocarditis poses a challenge to treat; is difficult to eradicate with pharmacologic therapy alone, and usually requires surgical intervention.[15,18,31] Most of these patients have multiple comorbidities and are difficult to operate on, making treatment further demanding. According to the Infectious Diseases Society of America (IDSA) guidelines,[15] native valve candida endocarditis should be treated with lipid formulation amphotericin B, with or without flucytosine, or with high-dose echinocandin. Valve replacement for native and prosthetic valve is recommended followed by at least 6 weeks of antifungal therapy, if surgical intervention is possible; otherwise long-term suppressive therapy with fluconazole is recommended.[15] However, it should be noted that there are no clinical trials evaluating the best approach in these cases due to their rarity. There is nonetheless a prevailing opinion that the best approach is a prolonged combination antifungal therapy until clearing of the infection followed by surgical intervention and suppressive antifungal therapy.[31] According to a comparative literature review, spanning a 12-year period by Garzoni et al., 58% of patients with candida endocarditis received combined medical and surgical management and most cases involved native valves (72.4%). Mortality was lower when surgical intervention was combined with medical therapy.[18] Another meta-analysis also suggested that combined surgical and medical treatment was associated with a lower mortality rate.[10] A report by Kan et al. suggested that initial aggressive medical therapy followed by valve debridement and prolonged course of postoperative oral antifungal therapy had better success rates.[14]

Despite her delicate condition, our patient received optimal management. She underwent surgical resection of the vegetation and valvuloplasty after receiving 9 weeks of combination therapy followed by another 6 weeks of treatment. She was also discharged on suppressive therapy with fluconazole but unfortunately passed away 1 week after discharge due to cardiac arrest likely related to aspiration.

CONCLUSION

Invasive candida infections pose a serious threat in hospitalized and debilitated pediatric patients. *C. parapsilosis* is a significant emerging nosocomial pathogen. Candidemia could lead to fungal endocarditis in certain high-risk groups that leads to an even higher mortality rate. Although there is no clear consensus based on clinical trials regarding the optimal management approach to these cases, present guidelines suggest combined medical and surgical intervention with a prolonged antifungal suppressive therapy in selected patients.

QUESTIONS

1. What are the major risk factors for invasive candidiasis?

2. What makes *Candida parapsilosis* an important nosocomial pathogen?

3. What are the risk factors for fungal endocarditis?

4. Describe the optimal treatment plan for candida endocarditis.

5. Discuss possible preventive strategies to reduce risk for invasive candidiasis.

REFERENCES

1. Barberino MG, Silva N, Reboucas C, et al. Evaluation of blood stream infections by Candida in three tertiary hospitals in Salvador, Brazil: a case-control study. *Braz J Infect Dis* 2006,10(1).36–40.

2. Rodriguez D, Almirante B, Park BJ, et al. Candidemia in neonatal intensive care units: Barcelona, Spain. *Pediatr Infect Dis J.* 2006;25(3):224–229.

3. San Miguel LG, Cobo J, Otheo E, et al. Candidemia in pediatric patients with congenital heart disease. *Diagn Microbiol Infecti Dis* 2006;55(3):203–207.

4. Pfaller MA, Diekema DJ. Epidemiology of invasive candidiasis: a persistent public health problem. *Clin Microbiol Rev* 2007;20(1):133–63.

5. Conde-Rosa A, Amador R, Perez-Torres D, et al. Candidemia distribution, associated risk factors, and attributed mortality at a university-based medical center. *Puerto Rico Health Sci J* 2010;29(1):26–29.

6. Steinbach WJ. Pediatric invasive candidiasis: epidemiology and diagnosis in children. *J Fungi* 2016;2(5).

7. Singhi S, Deep A. Invasive candidiasis in pediatric intensive care units. *Indian J Pediatr* 2009;76(10):1033–1044.

8. Trofa D, Gacser A, Nosanchuk JD. *Candida parapsilosis*, an emerging fungal pathogen. *Clin Microbiol Rev* 2008;21(4):606–625.

9. Pammi M, Holland L, Butler G, Gacser A, Bliss JM. *Candida parapsilosis* is a significant neonatal pathogen: a systematic review and meta-analysis. *Pediatr Infect Dis J* 2013;32(5):e206–e216.

10. Steinbach WJ, Perfect JR, Cabell CH, et al. A meta-analysis of medical versus surgical therapy for Candida endocarditis. *J Infect* 2005;51(3):230–247.

11. Grim SA, Berger K, Teng C, et al. Timing of susceptibility-based antifungal drug administration in patients with Candida bloodstream infection: correlation with outcomes. *J Antimicrob Chemother* 2012;67(3):707–714.

12. Ankhi Dutta TEZ, Debra L. Palazzi. An update on the epidemiology of Candidemia in children. *Curr Fungal Infect Rep* 2012;6(4).

13. Toyoda S, Tajima E, Fukuda R, et al. Early surgical intervention and optimal medical treatment for *Candida parapsilosis* endocarditis. *Intern Med* 2015;54(4):411–413.

14. Kan CD, Luo CY, Lin PY, Yang YJ. Native-valve endocarditis due to *Candida parapsilosis*. *Interact Cardiovasc Thorac Surg* 2002;1(2):66–68.

15. Pappas PG, Kauffman CA, Andes DR, et al. Clinical practice guideline for the management of Candidiasis: 2016 update by the Infectious Diseases Society of America. *Clin Infect Dis* 2016;62(4):e1–e50.

16. Shokohi T, Nouraei SM, Afsarian MH, Najafi N, Mehdipour S. Fungal prosthetic valve endocarditis by *Candida parapsilosis*: a case report. *Jundishapur J Microbiol* 2014;7(3):e9428.

17. Gullu AU, Akcar M, Arnaz A, Kizilay M. Candida parapsilosis tricuspid native valve endocarditis: 3-year follow-up after surgical treatment. *Interact Cardiovasc Thorac Surg* 2008;7(3):513–514.

18. Garzoni C, Nobre VA, Garbino J. *Candida parapsilosis* endocarditis: a comparative review of the literature. *Eur J Clin MicrobiolInfect Dis* 2007;26(12):915–926.

19. Mvondo CM, D'Auria F, Sordillo P, Pellegrino A, Adreoni M, Chiariello L. *Candida parapsilosis* endocarditis on a prosthetic aortic valve with unclear echocardiographic features. *Cardiovasc J Africa* 2013;24(3):e7–e8.

20. Lee CS, Choi JB, Kim KH. *Candida parapsilosis* bioprosthetic valve endocarditis inducing aortic valve stenosis. *Texas Heart Inst J*2013;40(4):502–504.

21. Silva-Pinto A, Ferraz R, Casanova J, Sarmento A, Santos L. *Candida parapsilosis* prosthetic valve endocarditis. *Med Mycol Case Rep* 2015;9:37–38.

22. Wallner M, Steyer G, Krause R, Gstettner C, von Lewinski D. Fungal endocarditis of a bioprosthetic aortic valve. Pharmacological treatment of a *Candida parapsilosis* endocarditis. *Herz* 2013;38(4):431–434.

23. Dotis J, Prasad PA, Zaoutis T, Roilides E. Epidemiology, risk factors and outcome of *Candida parapsilosis* bloodstream infection in children. *Pediatr Infect Dis J* 2012;31(6):557–560.

24. Sutcu M, Salman N, Akturk H, et al. Epidemiologic and microbiologic evaluation of nosocomial infections associated with *Candida spp.* in children: a multicenter study from Istanbul, Turkey. *Am J Infect Control*. 2016 Oct 1;44(10):1139-1143. doi: 10.1016/j.ajic.2016.03.056.

25. Singh R, Parija SC. *Candida parapsilosis* : an emerging fungal pathogen. *Indian J Med Res* 2012;136(4): 671–673.

26. Celebi S, Hacimustafaoglu M, Ozdemir O, Ozkaya G. Nosocomial candidaemia in children: results of a 9-year study. *Mycoses* 2008;51(3):248–257.

27. Kuhn DM, Mikherjee PK, Clark TA, et al. *Candida parapsilosis* characterization in an outbreak setting. *Emerging Infectious Diseases* 2004;10(6):1074–1081.

28. Nucci M. Persistent candidemia: causes and investigations. *Curr Fungal Infect Rep* 2011;5(1):3–11.

29. Chakrabarti C, Sood SK, Parnell V, Rubin LG. Prolonged candidemia in infants following surgery for congenital heart disease. *Infect Control Hosp Epidemiol* 2003;24(10):753–757.

30. Chae YT, Jeong SJ, Ku NS, et al. Risk factors and prognosis for persistent candidemia without catheter colonization. *Infect Chemother* 2012;44(1):44.

31. Baddour LM, Wilson WR, Bayer AS, et al. Infective endocarditis in adults: diagnosis, antimicrobial therapy, and management of complications: a scientific statement for healthcare professionals from the American Heart Association. *Circulation* 2015;132(15):1435–1486.

32. Pierrotti LC, Baddour LM. Fungal endocarditis, 1995-2000. *Chest* 2002;122(1):302–310.

33. Gilani AA, Barr CS. Recurrent *Candida parapsilosis* infective endocarditis aortic root replacement. *Br J Hosp Med* 2012;73(8):468–469.

Chapter 11

Considerations in Clinical Microbiology Testing and Reporting

Ziad Daoud, Roukoz A. Karam, and Khalil Masri

ABSTRACT

The clinical microbiology laboratory plays a critical role in the diagnosis and treatment of infectious diseases, as well as in infection control and antimicrobial stewardship. Classically, bacterial isolates are tested versus a panel of antibiotics representing different families and categories to determine the phenotypic profile of resistance. Interpretation of bacterial growth in the presence of antibiotics (as minimum inhibitory concentrations or inhibition diameters) is done according to international guidelines (such as Clinical Laboratory Standards Institute [CLSI] and the European Committee on Antimicrobial Susceptibility Testing [EUCAST] breakpoints) that are updated on an annual basis. In view of the complexity of the mechanisms of resistance as well as the advances in detection, interpretation, and reporting of the profile of resistance, microbiologists should be aware and up to date about the latest developments in this field, and techniques should be continuously upgraded in order to meet the most recent and most reliable standard. A misinterpreted result means a wrong treatment for the patient.

INTRODUCTION

The phenomenon of antimicrobial resistance is constantly increasing at both national and international levels.[1,2] Unfortunately, the development of new antimicrobials is not coping with this increase, and there is no expectation of development of new molecules in the near future.[3] In this context, understanding, detecting, and reporting of resistance in clinical isolates is of vital importance for the patient and the future of resistance.

When talking about the usefulness of a susceptibility report for the clinician, the first concept to address is the relevance of the antibiotic susceptibility testing in terms of technique and interpretation. This should be considered as the intersection of multiple concepts that are integrated to provide a suggestion about an antimicrobial activity on a particular pathogen present in a particular anatomic site. For a proper understanding of this, the knowledge of the mechanisms of bacterial resistance, as well as the pharmacokinetic/pharmacodynamic parameters of antibacterial agents becomes a must. All this should lead to appropriate reading, analysis, interpretation, and reporting of the susceptibility testing.

We review here some important aspects of antibiotic susceptibility testing through two clinical cases.

CLINICAL CASE 1

The patient was a 76-year-old male with past medical history of type 2 diabetes mellitus with hypertension, temporal arteritis, cerebrovascular accident, and heart failure. The patient was admitted 2 months ago for sepsis secondary to lung abscess. He was treated with amoxicillin–clavulanic acid for *Streptococcus spp.* isolated from blood; a urinary Foley catheter was inserted and was kept for 5 days because of acute kidney injury. The patient improved clinically and was subsequently discharged.

He was admitted 2 months later for fever chills and dysuria that started 2 days prior to admission. On physical examination, the patient was well oriented, with left hemiparesis. The lungs were clear and the abdomen was soft. Pain and dullness were reported on the suprapubic area.

Blood test creatinine was 12 mg/L, electrolytes normal, white blood cells 18,000, and C-reactive protein (CRP) level 113 mg/mL. Urinalysis reported presence of bacteria and white blood cells (WBC) count of 80–90. Urine culture yielded an extended spectrum beta-lactamase (ESBL) producing *Escherichia* coli with a typical pattern of resistance to cephalosporins including resistance to all first, second, third, and fourth generations. The patient was therefore put on imipenem (500 mg every 8 h).

At the microbiological level, the antibiotic susceptibility testing (Kirby–Bauer technique) showed narrow diameters of inhibition around cephalosporin discs with the exception of cefepime that showed a diameter of 27 mm (Fig. 11.1). An interpretive reading was done, and the organism was reported as resistant to cefepime accordingly.

So, How Accurate Was This Reporting?

The classification and understanding of the role of β-lactamases is increasingly complex and ESBLs have added a new point of complexity that has forced microbiology laboratories to

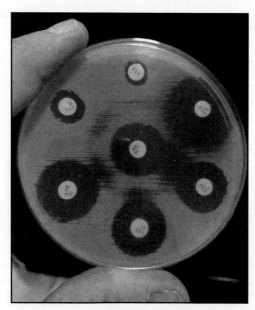

FIGURE 11.1 ESBL-producing *E.coli* (Case 1).

modify some behaviors to achieve good detection of these enzymes.[4] They can be seen in any *Enterobacteria*, commonly in *E. coli* and *Klebsiella spp*. They vary in frequency from one center to another, and even between different wards in the same institution. It is very important to monitor their occurrence and epidemiology; microbiology labs should carefully report these organisms. Classically, microbiologists detect ESBL production using a special sketch of antibiotic discs that allows the production of a specific keyhole effect between clavulanic acid and third/fourth generation cephalosporins. When this induced synergy is observed and the organism is subsequently labeled as ESBL, the organism is reported as intermediate or resistant to all cephalosporins.[5]

In 2014,[6] a new category called susceptible-dose dependent (SDD) was adopted for cefepime by the Clinical and Laboratory Standards Institute (CLSI) subcommittee on antimicrobial susceptibility testing. The resistance interpretive criteria were revised therefore, and new breakpoints were approved. The previous susceptibility criteria (2013 and before) included an MIC $\leq$ 8 mcg/mL and an inhibition diameter of $\geq$18 mm. Intermediate range corresponded to an MIC of 16 mcg/mL and to diameters between 15 and 17 mm, whereas resistance criteria included an MIC $\geq$ 32 mcg/mL and a diameter of inhibition $\leq$ 14 mm.[6] The revised 2014 recommendations defined susceptible strains with MICs $\leq$ 2 mcg/mL and diameters $\geq$ 25 mm, a new category "susceptible-dose dependent" with MICs between 4 and 8 mcg/mL and diameters of 19–24 mm, and resistance for MICs $\geq$ 16 mcg/mL and diameters $\leq$ 18 mm.

This change was suggested by three main factors: (1) the 2013 and older breakpoints take into consideration a dose of cefepime that is higher than the one often used, (2) the treatment of isolates showing an MIC of 4 mcg/mL or 8 mcg/mL with cefepime led to unexpected clinical failures. This was clear with treatment regimens using lower doses of this antibiotic, (3) the unavailability of new drugs for the near future with potential activity on multidrug-resistant Gram-negative bacteria and the spread of mechanisms of resistance among these organisms.

SDD adoption is considered a new approach to interpret susceptibility of antibacterial agents; however, this category has been used for antifungal susceptibility testing interpretation. This new category infers that the dosing regimen used in a specific patient is a major determinant of efficiency of the antibacterial agent in question, and subsequently will reflect on the susceptibility of the bacterial isolate. For clinical success, it becomes necessary to implement higher and/or more frequent doses exposing, therefore, the pathogen to higher concentrations of antibiotics than the ones used in establishing the susceptible area, in cases where MIC determination or disc diffusion method (Kirby–Bauer) suggests an SDD.

To be on the safe side and to achieve the highest possibility of appropriate treatment of an SDD isolate, the maximum approved concentration of cefepime should be considered. The application of SDD category in cefepime breakpoints replaces the "intermediate" category definition for antibacterial agents when reporting susceptibility results of this antibiotic for enterobacteriaceae (MIC = 4 or 8 mcg/mL or inhibition diameter = 19–24 mm). This is possible in view of the many dosing regimen options approved for cefepime.[6]

The introduction of the new concept of SDD came after the adoption of new cutoff values (breakpoints) that reduced the diameters of susceptibility around 3rd and 4th generation cephalosporins. It is no more recommended to amend the results of susceptibility around these antibiotics, but to report them as measured. In 2010, the CLSI revised the breakpoints of cephalosporins and cephamycins and recommended that there is no need to perform routine ESBL testing. This was emphasized with the new cefepime breakpoints and now, ESBL testing takes only an epidemiological and infection control dimension rather than reporting importance.

The inclusion of the SDD category is expected to refine susceptibility, to encourage clinicians to consider the possibility of using cefepime for treatment of ESBLs, and to increase the awareness of antibiotic stewardship programs about the appropriate use of antibiotics.

In cases of SDD reporting, it is advisable to:

1. Meet with the antimicrobial stewardship committees, infectious diseases practitioners, clinical pharmacists, etc. and inform them of these changes, and adapt the laboratory information system (LIS) accordingly.
2. Include an explanatory note about SDD. CLSI recommends the following: *"The interpretive criterion for susceptible is based on a dosage regimen of 1 g every 12 h. The interpretive criterion for susceptible-dose dependent is based on dosing regimens that result in higher cefepime exposure, either higher doses or more frequent doses or both, up to approved maximum dosing regimens".*

It is worth noting that this new designation is currently applied exclusively for cefepime versus enterobacteriaceae. The CLSI is examining the possibility for more combinations of antibiotic/bacteria where multiple dosing options are recommended. The SDD category does not depend on the patient or the specimen.[6]

CLINICAL CASE 2

A 42-year-old female with past medical history of recurrent right ear infection was admitted on September 30, 2016, with vertigo, right ear pain, and purulent secretions. The history goes back to many years ago when she started to have recurrent otitis media and received antibiotics on multiple occasions.

The patient was seen by an ear, nose, and throat (ENT) physician, few weeks ago before admission for ear effusion and secretions. She was given, among other antibiotics, amoxicillin–clavulanic acid for 2 weeks, then was switched to ciprofloxacin without clinical improvement.

On admission, the patient was conscious and oriented, her lung and abdominal examinations were normal. The ENT examination showed perforated tympanic membrane on the right side with purulent effusion. Her blood sugar was 0.85 g/L, creatinine 8 mg/L, and CRP level 12 mg/mL. White blood cells count was 7,630 white blood cells per microliter, Hemoglobin was 13,8 g/dL and platelets 241,000. The chest X-ray was normal. The CT scan reported a temporal bone interruption of the right tympanic membrane with soft tissue thickening along the right middle ear cavity and right mastoid air cells, suggestive of otitis media, and possible acute mastoiditis. Bacteriology culture of ear secretions reported a *Pseudomonas aeruginosa* resistant to carbapenems, intermediate to cefepime and ceftazidime, and susceptible to colistin.

The patient was put on cefepime (2 g i.v. every 8 h) in addition to colistin (3 million units every 8 h). Clinically, a significant improvement was observed, reflected by decreased ear pain and absence of secretions.

A closer look at the antibiotic testing results revealed that the organism showed a diameter of inhibition of 28 mm around the imipenem disc with total absence of inhibition around meropenem disc (Fig. 11.2). This result was reported as resistant to both antibiotics to avoid giving the physician any possibility of false impression of safety in using imipenem for treatment.

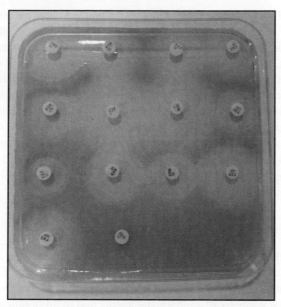

FIGURE 11.2   *Pseudomonas aeruginosa* susceptible to imipenem and resistant to meropenem (Case 2).

So, How Correct Was This Reporting?

When analyzing this susceptibility, it is important to consider that the discordance of in vitro susceptibility to meropenem versus imipenem is real. *P. aeruginosa* is a pathogen with natural resistance to various antimicrobial agents. The association of different types of drug efflux pumps and different degrees of outer membrane permeability result in an exceptional intrinsic resistance in *Pseudomonas*.

On the basis of patterns of resistance and susceptibility to carbapenems, clinical isolates of carbapenem-resistant *P. aeruginosa* can be divided into three groups: (1) IRMS (imipenem resistant meropenem susceptible group), (2) ISMR (imipenem susceptible meropenem resistant) group, and (3) IRMR (imipenem resistant meropenem resistant) group.[7–9] This variability suggests resistance to carbapenem; in *Pseudomonas,* it is due to several mechanisms in concert. In the absence of carbapenem-hydrolyzing enzymes, mainly metallo-beta-lactamases (MBLs), carbapenem resistance is usually multifactorial. Most commonly, the mechanisms of resistance include: the presence of OprD, expressions of the MexAB–OprM and the MexEF–OprN systems, and the production of β-lactamases including carbapenemases, such as MBLs.[10]

Studies that addressed this issue showed that resistance to carbapenems is mostly mediated by OprD loss. This mainly confers resistance to imipenem coupled with a low-grade resistance to meropenem.[8,9] On the other hand, multidrug efflux systems can play an important role in this context, contributing to carbapenem resistance (in addition to mediating resistance to quinolone, chloramphenicol, and other antibiotics).

Strains overexpressing the MexAB–OprM system exhibit carbapenem resistance by pumping the drug out. Those expressing the MexEF–OprN system confer carbapenem resistance by repressing the transcription of OprD,[11,12] whereas strains that express MexCE–OprJ (NfxB mutants) become more susceptible to imipenem.[13]

In addition to all this, chromosomal AmpC β-lactamase plays an important role in carbapenem resistance in *P. aeruginosa*, mainly when it is coupled to other mechanisms of resistance.[14] It is true that loss of OprD, efflux systems, and β-lactamases have been well identified in the lab; however, their mutualistic activity in vivo remains difficult to predict.

In the absence of a strict CLSI or European Committee on Antimicrobial Susceptibility Testing (EUCAST) recommendation to amend the susceptibility to imipenem and resistance to meropenem in clinical isolates of *P. aeruginosa*, the clinical microbiologist faces a challenge in reporting this resistance. It is advisable always to initiate a discussion with the clinician about this matter or to include a note along with the reporting of such results. In all cases, it is a must to test both antibiotics (imipenem and meropenem) with *Pseudomonas* isolates, since the profile of resistance will vary with the specific mechanisms that makes the reporting problematic.

QUESTIONS

1. Give one main change that was introduced to the CLSI guidelines in 2014 concerning interpretation of resistance of ESBL-producing enterobacteriaceae. Discuss.
2. What does the category SDD mean with antibacterial agents interpretation of susceptibility testing? Does it apply to all antibacterial agents and to all organisms?
3. What is the clinical value of adding meropenem and imipenem to the antibiotic testing formulary in the clinical microbiology lab?
4. What are the mechanisms of resistance of *Pseudomonas* to carbapenems in the context of beta-lactamases?
5. How does clinical microbiology integrate in infectious diseases? What are the drawbacks of microbiology lab misinterpretation of results on the patient?

REFERENCES

1. de Kraker MEA, Jarlier V, Monen JCM, Heuer OE, van de Sande N, Grundmann H. The changing epidemiology of bacteraemias in Europe: trends from the European Antimicrobial Resistance Surveillance System. *Clin Microbio Inf* 2013, 19(9):860–868.
2. Smith Richard, Coast Joanna. The true cost of antimicrobial resistance. *BMJ* 2013; 346:1497.
3. Ian M Gould and Abhijit M Bal. New antibiotic agents in the pipeline and how they can help overcome microbial resistance, *Virulence* 2013. 4(2).
4. Bush K. Proliferation and significance of clinically relevant β-lactamases. *Ann NY Acad Sci* 2013; 1277: 84–90.
5. CLSI. Performance Standards for Antimicrobial Susceptibility Testing: 20th Informational Supplement, CLSI Document M100-S20. Wayne, PA: Clinical and Laboratory Standards Institute; 2010.
6. CLSI. Performance Standards for Antimicrobial Susceptibility Testing: 24th Informational Supplement, CLSI Document M100-S24. Wayne, PA: Clinical and Laboratory Standards Institute; 2014.
7. Meletis G, Exindari M, Vavatsi N, Sofianou D, Diza E. Mechanisms responsible for the emergence of carbapenem resistance in *Pseudomonas aeruginosa*. *Hippokratia*. 2012;16(4):303–307.
8. Fernández L, Hancock REW. Adaptive and mutational resistance: role of porins and efflux pumps in drug resistance. *Clin Microbiol Rev.* 2012;25(4):661–681. doi:10.1128/CMR.00043–12.
9. Camila Rizek, Liang Fu, Leticia Cavalcanti dos Santos, et al. Characterization of carbapenem-resistant *Pseudomonas aeruginosa* clinical isolates, carrying multiple genes coding for this antibiotic resistance. *Ann Clin Microbiol Antimicrob* 2014, 13:43.
10. Ester Fuste, Lidia Lopez-Jimenez, Concha Segura, Eusebio Gainza, Teresa Vinuesa, Miguel Vinas. Carbapenem-resistance mechanisms of multidrug-resistant *Pseudomonas aeruginosa*. *J Med Microbiol* (2013), 62:1317–1325.

11. Ochs MM, McCusker MP, Bains M, Hancock RE. Negative regulation of the *Pseudomonas aeruginosa* outer membrane porin OprD selective for imipenem and basic amino acids. *Antimicrob Agents Chemother.* 1999; 43(5):1085–1090.

12. Maseda H, Yoneyama H, Nakae T. Assignment of the substrate-selective subunits of the MexEF-OprN multidrug efflux pump of *Pseudomonas aeruginosa*. *Antimicrob Agents Chemother.* 2000; 44(3):658–664.

13. Masuda N, Gotoh N, Ohya S, Nishino T. Quantitative correlation between susceptibility and OprJ production in NfxB mutants of *Pseudomonas aeruginosa*. *Antimicrob Agents Chemother.* 1996 Apr; 40(4):909–913.

14. Masuda N, Gotoh N, Ishii C I, Sakagawa E, Ohya S, Nishino T. Interplay between chromosomal β-lactamase and the MexAB-OprM efflux system in intrinsic resistance to β-lactamas in *Pseudomonas aeruginosa*. *Antimicrob Agents Chemother.* 1999;43:400–402.

Chapter 12

Myocarditis in Toxocariasis: Case Report and Review of the Literature

Nesrine Rizk, Amer Toutonji, Abdallah Rebeiz, and Hiba El Hajj

ABSTRACT

Eosinophilic myocarditis is a rare cardiac disease characterized by heart muscle inflammation due to eosinophilic infiltration. Eosinophilic myocarditis can be a manifestation of toxocariasis, a parasitic infection caused by the zoonotic ascarids *Toxocara canis* and *Toxocara cati*. In both its acute and chronic forms, eosinophilic myocarditis can be life-threatening and warrants prompt treatment with systemic steroids.

In this chapter, we report the first case of eosinophilic myocarditis in Lebanon as a result of infection with *Toxocara canis*. The patient was a 41-year-old man who presented with acute onset of left-sided chest pain associated with nausea, dizziness, and dyspnea, and preceded by a 2-week history of high-grade fever and myalgias. On presentation, the patient was found to be fatigued and pale. He had bilateral wheezes and fine basilar crackles on lung auscultation. There were no cardiac murmurs and his abdomen was obese and nontender. He underwent cardiac catheterization that revealed normal coronaries and severe global hypokynesis. The echocardiogram revealed myocardial hypertrophy. A computed tomography (CT) scan of the chest revealed diffuse bilateral nodular opacities with the largest in the left lower lobe and mediastinal lymphadenopathy. The eosinophilic count increased to 5049 cells/mm^3. Cardiac magnetic resonance imaging (MRI) showed an increased left ventricle (LV) wall thickness, mildly reduced systolic function (EF 49%), and a small pericardial effusion without hemodynamic significance. Serologic testing for systemic parasitic infections revealed toxocariais. This chapter provides an overview of the rare published case reports of *Toxacara* related EM and presents the first related case in Lebanon.

PATIENT CASE PRESENTATION

This is the case of a 41-year-old man who presented on June 20, 2014 at the American University of Beirut Medical Center (AUBMC) Emergency Department with acute onset of left-sided chest pain, associated with nausea, dizziness, and dyspnea. Acute coronary syndrome was suspected on the basis of finding ST segment depression on the electrocardiogram (ECG) and elevated troponin and cardiac markers in the serum.

The patient lived and worked in Guinea in West Africa; he had returned to Lebanon a month prior to this presentation. The current symptoms were preceded by a 2-week history of high-grade fever and myalgias, treated with different antibiotics and antimalarial agents to no avail. He denied any outdoor activities in Guinea, stating that he spent most of his time

72

in an office. He had no previous medical problems, except for hypercholesterolemia and malaria treated in 2008. He was married; his wife and children lived in Lebanon. He visited his family several times per year. He was a heavy smoker, and denied heavy alcohol use. He had no pets at home.

On presentation to our hospital, his body temperature was 37°C, his blood pressure was 102/76 mm Hg, and heart rate was 98 beats per minute. He was found to be fatigued and pale. There was no jaundice and no icterus; he had bilateral wheezes and fine basilar crackles on lung auscultation. There were no cardiac murmurs and his abdomen was obese and nontender. Therapy with antiplatelet agents was started and the patient was admitted to the CCU for monitoring. The following laboratory findings were obtained initially: white blood cell count of 17,200 per mm^3, eosinophils 15% (2580 cells/mm^3), C-reactive protein level 29 mg/L, ESR 20 mm/h. The next day, he underwent cardiac catheterization that revealed normal coronaries and decreased wall motion; but the echocardiogram revealed myocardial thickening. On the second night of his hospitalization, he developed a cough and a fever of 39°C. A CT scan of the chest revealed diffuse bilateral nodular opacities with the largest in the left lower lobe and mediastinal lymphadenopathy. The eosinophilic count increased to 5049 cells/mm^3. Cardiac MRI showed an increased LV wall thickness, mildly reduced systolic function (EF 49%), and a small pericardial effusion without hemodynamic significance (Fig. 12.1). On the basis of these findings, we suspected eosinophilic myocarditis (EM).

The patient was started on diuresis and treatment for the heart failure with noticeable improvement as the dyspnea and the fever resolved on the third day. He was discharged home on albendazole for 6 weeks and diuretics as well as beta-blockers and tritace. Serologic testing for systemic parasitic infections revealed toxocariais with *Toxocara canis* IgG/EIA of 14.0 U/mL and IgM-positive reaction with specific parasitic antigens. The patient was seen several weeks later for follow-up. He reported continued improvement and complete resolution of the dyspnea and cough. Unfortunately, we could not repeat the serologic titers.

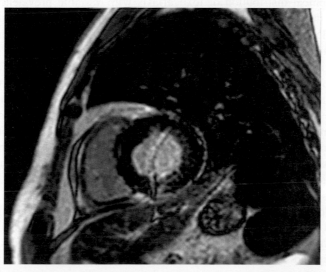

FIGURE 12.1 Cardiac magnetic resonance showing evidence of a focal area of myocarditis in the left ventricle right at the right ventricle insertion point.

CASE DISCUSSION AND OVERVIEW OF THE LITERATURE

EM is a rare cardiac disease characterized by heart muscle inflammation due to eosinophilic infiltration. In both its acute and chronic forms, EM can be life-threatening and warrants prompt treatment with systemic steroids.[1] Reported etiologies in the literature mainly include autoimmune diseases, parasitic infections, and hypersensitivity to drugs and vaccinations.[2–5] So far, only seven cases of EM have been associated with toxocariasis, a parasitic infection[1,2,6–9] (Table 12.1) caused by the zoonotic ascarids *T. canis* and *T. cati*. In this chapter, we report the first case of EM in Lebanon as a result of infection with *T. canis*.

PATHOGENESIS

Life Cycle

The life cycle of *T. canis* and *T. cati* starts in their definitive hosts, canids, and felids, respectively. Female worms in the upper digestive tract produce thousands of eggs per day; these eggs are passed in the feces to the environment, where they embryonate and become infective under appropriate conditions of temperature.[10] Embryonated eggs can persist in the soil for years until they are either ingested by their definitive hosts or by paratenic hosts like humans. In definitive hosts, the eggs hatch and the larvae mature in the upper digestive system, lay eggs and release them in feces, and restart the cycle. However, if ingested by humans, the eggs hatch but the small larvae are incapable of maturation beyond the second-stage, and instead, penetrate the intestinal wall and are carried by the circulation to a wide variety of tissues (liver, heart, lungs, brain, muscle, eyes) causing damage to the organs.[11]

Epidemiology

The analysis of human seroprevalence data from studies done in many countries reflects a wide geographical distribution of toxocariasis with variable prevalence between and within each of the countries.[12,13] For instance, seroprevalence in Ghana and the Republic of Marshall Islands exceeds 50%,[14,15] whereas within Venezuela and Poland, it ranges from < 10% to > 60%.[16,17] In the USA and Iran, the seroprevalence are 13.9% and 15.8%, respectively.[18,19] Seroprevalence studies were also done in Japan, Korea, Indonesia, Turkey, Slovakia, Brazil, Mexico, and other countries and indicate a probable increase in the seroprevalence trend.[13,20–24] It is important, however, to recognize the limitations of seroprevalence studies: the selected samples range between preschoolers, school students, and adults from selected regions within the countries and are probably not be representative of the whole population.[11] In addition, immunologic diagnostic techniques used to determine the seroprevalence of *T. canis* might cross-react with other parasites leading to an overestimation.[25]

Nonetheless, the global prevalence of toxocariasis seen in these preliminary seroprevalence data can probably be explained by the high (>20%) incidence of dog and cat infections with adult *Toxocara* worms in Western countries[10] and the high level of contamination of outdoor parks and backyards of homes with *Toxocara* eggs from pet feces.[26,27] In addition to pet ownership and soil contamination by animal feces, other risk factors for toxocariasis including African–American race, poverty, male sex, geophagia amongst children and eating raw meat, and vegetables have also been cited.[23,28–31]

TABLE 12.1 Summary of All Case Reports of Toxocariasis with Cardiac Involvement.

Case	Country	Sex/Age (years)	Heart Pathology	Endomyocardial Biopsy (EMB)	Peripheral Eosinophil Count (/µL)	Serum Total IgE (IU/mL)	Risk Factors	Other Tests
1[1]	Japan	M/27	Thick edematous LV + eosinophilic PE (3264/µL)	Eosinophilic infiltration, some lymphocytes and focal myocyte necrosis	Mildly elevated (not specified)	662	Raw deer meat	Exclusion of myocarditis-causing viruses, collagen disease, drug-induced and radiation-induced myocarditis
2[2]	Japan	M/26	Thick LV + PE		26,000		Raw meat	Exclusion of myocarditis-causing viruses
3[39]	Korea	M/72	Concentric LV hypertrophy + PE		2340	419	Raw cow liver	ECP = 20.9 mcg/L
4[39]	Korea	M/45	Thick edematous LV + PE		4453	532		ECP = 57.2 mcg/L
5[9]	Korea	M/57	Right heart failure + thick right ventricular apex + RA thrombus	No evidence of eosinophilic infiltration	1,410 (persisted for 8 months)	5,000	Dog owner	Elevated IgG; pericardiotomy followed by biopsy showed non-specific pericarditis
6[7]	Korea	F/41	Thick edematous LV	Myocyte necrosis and degeneration	8430		None – raw vegetables?	
7[6]	Japan	M/19	Thick LV + PE	Eosinophilic inflammation, interstitial edema and myocyte necrosis	1053		Raw deer meat	ECP = 54.9; active viral infections were ruled out

Note: ECP, eosinophil cationic protein; LV, left ventricle; PE, pericardial effusion; RA, right atrium.

Clinical Course

Toxocariasis in humans can be asymptomatic and self-limiting but it can also present clinically with mild to severe organ injury. Mild organ injury is seen in "covert toxocariasis" and "common toxocariasis" that have been respectively identified in case–control studies in seropositive children in Ireland[32] and in French adults.[33] Severe toxocariasis is caused by the migration of second-stage larvae through body tissues leading to inflammation, which can be limited to the eyes and optic nerves causing visual symptoms as in ocular larva migrans (OLM) or can affect visceral organs as in visceral larva migrans (VLM).[10]

VLM typically occurs in young children due to infection with embryonated eggs of *T. canis* from eating dirt and exposure to puppies that have not been dewormed.[10,34] It most often damages the liver and lungs, but has also been reported in the CNS, kidney, and heart.[10,23,35] It is also of importance that a concomitant remarkable eosinophilia is usually present in peripheral blood and/or on biopsy of the affected organs.[11]

DIAGNOSIS

The case definition for inclusion was based on clinical symptoms in accordance with cardiac disease and one of the following criteria:

(A) Detection of: (i) parasite material or (ii) eosinophilic granuloma in histological sections of cardiac tissue or (iii) a shared environment with a dog or a cat with a confirmed *Toxocara spp.* infection.

(B) Cases fulfilling at least two of the following three criteria: (i) a positive serological titer, (ii) an increase or decrease of the titer during disease or treatment or (iii) eosinophilia ($>500/\mu L$).

Our patient fulfilled two criteria, as he did not perform the necessary blood testing to document a decreasing serologic titer. In this setting of high clinical suspicion, elevations of cardiac enzymes, electrocardiographic changes (nonspecific), echocardiography, and cardiac magnetic resonance imaging are helpful. Myocardial biopsy can provide a definitive diagnosis, but sampling errors limit its utility.

TREATMENT

There are currently no guidelines to dictate the choice of therapy and treatment course. It appears that a combination of antihelminthic and corticosteroids is the most frequently accepted, for a duration ranging from 1 week to 3 months. Supportive care and management of congestive heart failure symptoms are also necessary. There is no clear role for immunosuppressive therapy at this point. No objective means exist to evaluate success of treatment since parasite eradication in VLM patients cannot be assessed.[13,36,37] Albendazole (500 mg given twice daily for 5 days) is the currently recommended treatment for VLM.[8,36,37] Adjunct steroids are recommended for severe ocular involvement[13] and signs of systemic inflammation.

In the reviewed case reports, albendazole has been used in dosages of 200–1000 mg per day from 7 days up to 3 months. In two patients receiving an initial treatment for only 1–2 weeks, a second course had to be applied due to recurrence of symptoms.[38] Since cardiac toxocariasis is a potentially life-threatening disease, we suggest using higher doses (15 mg/kg or 800–1200 mg/day) and on the basis of the fact that none of the patients treated for more than 2–3 weeks had a relapse described, for a duration of at least 3–4 weeks. When giving albendazole for more than 3–4 weeks, the adverse events of albendazole—mainly hepatic toxicity and bone marrow suppression—have to be balanced against the potential benefits. The relevance of the additional use of corticosteroids seems less clear. Regimens ranging from steroids given from 3 days to up to several months have been used without clearly influencing the outcome. However, since the addition of corticosteroids can lead to a rapid improvement of symptoms,[2,6] this is advisable, especially in cases showing severe signs of systemic inflammation. We propose prednisone at a starting dose of 1 mg/kg body weight for 1 week. The consecutive tapering should be on the basis of clinical signs and symptoms and the eosinophil count. Treatment should be guided by close clinical and laboratory monitoring, including the eosinophil count and liver enzymes. A second course of antihelminthics and steroids may be necessary. Treatment of heart failure is according to the usual guidelines and is not in the scope of this article. The formation of a thrombus might occur as a complication of Loeffler's endocarditis and would demand anticoagulation.

CONCLUSION

We have described a case of a patient with *Toxocara* myocarditis for the first time in Lebanon. This patient could have acquired this parasitic infection in Lebanon, as toxocariais is endemic to this country. The definite diagnosis of *Toxocara* myocarditis should include a myocardial biopsy that proves the eosinophilic infiltration. This was not performed as our patient's condition improved significantly. It is important to consider *Toxocara* in the differential diagnosis of invasive systemic illnesses associated with eosinophilia.

QUESTIONS

1. What is the differential diagnosis of eosinophilic myocarditis?
2. List other forms of invasive toxocariasis. What are their causal agents?
3. How are the diagnostic criteria to be fulfilled to confirm a case of toxocariasis?
4. What is the treatment of toxocariasis? Is toxocariasis treatment always necessary with antiparasitic agents?
5. What is the approach to a patient with heart failure, dyspnea, and fever?

REFERENCES

1. Sangen H, Tanabe J, Takano H, Shimizu W. Successful early diagnosis and treatment in a case of *Toxocara canis*-induced eosinophilic myocarditis with eosinophil-rich pericardial effusion. *BMJ Case Rep.* 2015;2015.
2. Abe K, Shimokawa H, Kubota T, Nawa Y, Takeshita A. Myocarditis associated with visceral larva migrans due to *Toxocara canis*. *Intern Med.* 2002;41(9):706–708.
3. Barton M, Finkelstein Y, Opavsky MA, et al. Eosinophilic myocarditis temporally associated with conjugate meningococcal C and hepatitis B vaccines in children. *Pediatr Infect Dis J.* 2008;27(9):831–835.
4. Bilinska ZT, Bilinska M, Grzybowski J, et al. Unexpected eosinophilic myocarditis in a young woman with rapidly progressive dilated cardiomyopathy. *Int J Cardiol.* 2002;86(2–3):295–297.
5. Spry CJ, Take M, Tai PC. Eosinophilic disorders affecting the myocardium and endocardium: a review. *Heart Vessels Suppl.* 1985;1:240–242.
6. Enko K, Tada T, Ohgo KO, et al. Fulminant eosinophilic myocarditis associated with visceral larva migrans caused by *Toxocara canis* infection. *Circ J.* 2009;73(7):1344–1348

7. Kim JH, Chung WB, Chang KY, et al. Eosinophilic myocarditis associated with visceral larva migrans caused by *Toxocara canis* infection. *J Cardiovasc Ultrasound.* 2012;20(3):150–153.
8. Kuenzli E, Neumayr A, Chaney M, Blum J.Toxocariasis-associated cardiac diseases—A systematic review of the literature. *Acta Trop.* 2016;154:107–120.
9. Park HJ, You GI, Cho KI, et al. Cardiac involvement in hypereosinophilia associated with toxocariasis. *J Cardiovasc Ultrasound.* 2014;22(4): 224–227.
10. Magnaval JF, Glickman LT, Dorchies P, Morassin B. Highlights of human toxocariasis. *Korean J Parasitol.* 2001;39(1):1–11.
11. Nicoletti A, Toxocariasis. *Handb Clin Neurol,* 2013;114:217–228.
12. Macpherson CN. The epidemiology and public health importance of toxocariasis: a zoonosis of global importance. *Int J Parasitol.* 2013;43(12-13):999–1008.
13. Rubinsky-Elefant G, Hirata CE, Yamamoto JH, Ferreira MU. Human toxocariasis: diagnosis, worldwide seroprevalences and clinical expression of the systemic and ocular forms. *Ann Trop Med Parasitol.* 2010;104(1):3–23.
14. Fu CJ, Chuang TW, Lin HS, et al. Seroepidemiology of *Toxocara canis* infection among primary schoolchildren in the capital area of the Republic of the Marshall Islands. *BMC Infect Dis.* 2014;14:261.
15. Kyei G, Ayi I, Boampong JN, Turkson PK. Sero-epidemiology of *Toxocara Canis* infection in children attending four selected health facilities in the central region of Ghana. *Ghana Med J.* 2015;49(2):77–83.
16. Borecka A, Klapec T. Epidemiology of human toxocariasis in Poland – a review of cases 1978-2009. *Ann Agric Environ Med.* 2015;22(1):28–31.
17. Martinez M, García H, Figuera L, et al. Seroprevalence and risk factors of toxocariasis in preschool children in Aragua state, Venezuela. *Trans R Soc Trop Med Hyg.* 2015;109(9):579–588.
18. Abdi J, M Darabi, K Sayehmiri. Epidemiological situation of toxocariasis in Iran: meta-analysis and systematic review. *Pak J Biol Sci.* 2012;15(22):1052–1055.
19. Woodhall D.M, ML Eberhard, M.E. Parise, Neglected parasitic infections in the United States: toxocariasis. *Am J Trop Med Hyg.* 2014;90(5):810–813.
20. Akao N, Ohta N. Toxocariasis in Japan. *Parasitol Int.* 2007;56(2)87–93.
21. Dogan N, Dinleyici EC, Bor O, Töz SO, Ozbel Y. Seroepidemiological survey for *Toxocara canis* infection in the northwestern part of Turkey. *Turkiye Parazitol Derg.* 2007;31(4):288–291.
22. Hayashi E, Tuda J, Imada M, Akao N, Fujita K. The high prevalence of asymptomatic Toxocara infection among schoolchildren in Manado, Indonesia. *Southeast Asian J Trop Med Public Health.* 2005;36(6) 1399–1406.
23. Lee RM, Moore LB, Bottazzi ME, Hotez PJ. Toxocariasis in North America: a systematic review. *PLoS Negl Trop Dis.* 2014;8(8):e3116.
24. Oliart-Guzman H, Delfino BM, Martins AC, et al. Epidemiology and control of child toxocariasis in the western Brazilian Amazon – a population-based study. *Am J Trop Med Hyg.* 2014;90(4)670–681.
25. Rodriguez-Caballero A, Martínez-Gordillo MN, Medina-Flores Y, et al. Successful capture of *Toxocara canis* larva antigens from human serum samples. *Parasit Vectors.* 2015;8:264.
26. Capuano DM, M Rocha Gde. Environmental contamination by *Toxocara sp.* eggs in Ribeirao Preto, Sao Paulo State, Brazil. *Rev Inst Med Trop Sao Paulo.* 2005;47(4)223–226.
27. Jarosz W, Mizgajska-Wiktor H, Kirwan P, Konarski J, Rychlicki W, Wawrzyniak G. Developmental age, physical fitness and Toxocara seroprevalence amongst lower-secondary students living in rural areas contaminated with Toxocara eggs. *Parasitology.* 2010. 137(1)53–63.
28. Dutra GF, Pinto NS, de Avila LF, et al. Risk of infection by the consumption of liver of chickens inoculated with low doses of *Toxocara canis* eggs. *Vet Parasitol.* 2014;203(1-2)87–90.
29. Fellrath JM, JF Magnaval. Toxocariasis after slug ingestion characterized by severe neurologic, ocular, and pulmonary involvement. *Open Forum Infect Dis.* 2014;1(2):ofu063.
30. Noh Y, Hong ST, Yun JY, et al. Meningitis by *Toxocara canis* after ingestion of raw ostrich liver. *J Korean Med Sci.* 2012. 27(9):1105–1108.
31. Salem G, Schantz P. Toxocaral visceral larva migrans after ingestion of raw lamb liver. *Clin Infect Dis.* 1992;15(4):743–744.

32. Taylor MR, Keane CT, O'Connor P, Girdwood RW, Smith H. Clinical features of covert toxocariasis. *Scand J Infect Dis.* 1987;19(6):693–696.

33. Glickman LT, Magnaval JF, Domanski LM, et al. Visceral larva migrans in French adults: a new disease syndrome? *Am J Epidemiol.* 1987;125(6):1019–1034.

34. Nijsse R, Ploeger HW, Wagenaar JA, Mughini-Gras L. Toxocara canis in household dogs: prevalence, risk factors and owners' attitude towards deworming. *Parasitol Res.* 2015;114(2):561–569.

35. Chang S, Lim JH, Choi D, et al. Hepatic visceral larva migrans of *Toxocara canis*: CT and sonographic findings. *Am J Roentgenol.* 2006;187(6):W622–W629.

36. Ahn SJ, NK Ryoo, Woo SJ. Ocular toxocariasis: clinical features, diagnosis, treatment, and prevention. *Asia Pac Allergy.* 2014;4(3):134–141.

37. Ahn SJ, Woo SJ, Jin Y, et al. Clinical features and course of ocular toxocariasis in adults. *PLoS Negl Trop Dis.* 2014;8(6):e2938.

38. Despommier D. Toxocariasis: clinical aspects, epidemiology, medical ecology, and molecular aspects. *Clin Microbiol Rev.* 2003;16(2):265–272.

39. Sohn KH, Song WJ, Kim BK, et al. Eosinophilic myocarditis: case series and literature review. *Asia Pac Allergy.* 2015;5(2):123–127.

Chapter 13

Molecular Methods for Detection of Common Potentially Sexually Transmitted Bacterial Agents Causing Nonspecific Urogenital Infections

Asem A. Shehabi

ABSTRACT

Nonspecific urogenital infections caused mostly by *Chlamydia trachomatis*, *Mycoplasma genitalium*, and *Ureaplasma urealyticum* are difficult to diagnose by culture or serological methods in laboratories. Rapid and highly specific molecular methods are currently available for their laboratory diagnosis.

INTRODUCTION

Recently, the World Health Organization (WHO) and many other research studies have documented the increased prevalence of certain sexually transmitted bacterial agents as the cause of nonspecific urogenital infections and the development of various disease complications including infertility in females and males.[1–5] In particular, *Chlamydia trachomatis*, *Mycoplasma genitalium*, and *Ureaplasma urealyticum* are among the most prevalent potential bacterial pathogens found in the genital tract of humans with asymptomatic and symptomatic features.[2–5] Therefore, a rapid and accurate diagnosis of their presence in association with genital disease features requires administration of effective therapy to prevent their complications in the future.

Short descriptions of these fastidious bacterial agents and their rapid detection by molecular methods are given in the following sections.

Chlamydia trachomatis

This bacterium is one of the most frequent causes of sexually transmitted infections (STIs) in developed countries.[1,2,6] It is an obligate intracellular bacterium, which has a special biphasic developmental mechanism in infected tissues.[6] There are certain specific serovars associated with genitourinary tract infections, often causing diverse urogenital diseases, such as nonspecific urethritis, epididymitis, and proctitis in men, whereas causing cervicitis, urethritis, and pelvic inflammatory disease (PID) in women, and inclusion conjunctivitis and neonatal pneumonitis in infants through their infected mothers.[7] Other Chlamydia serovars L1, L2, L2a, and L3 that are found in the inguinal lymph nodes cause lymphogranuloma venereum (LGV); and most recently, type L2 is found frequently in human immunodeficiency virus-seropositive patients.[8] In general, between 50% and 70% of all *Chlamydia* genital infections among men and women can be asymptomatic and not diagnosed and treated.[6] In particular, *Chlamydia* infection in women may be associated with complications presented as Pelvic inflammatory disease (PID), ectopic pregnancy, and infertility.[7]

Laboratory Diagnosis

Cell culture of *C. trachomatis* has shown a very high specificity, but it is not useful for routine diagnosis of infection, since it lacks high sensitivity associated with collection of adequate specimens and technical difficulty in their transport and storage.[6] A laboratory diagnostic test can be best made using fresh urine specimen and PCR tests, since these tests have specificity and sensitivity and do not include invasive procedures for specimen collection.[3,9] DNA testing was the first molecular DNA test used for detection of *C. trachomatis*, and was mostly used before the introduction of PCR methods.[9] A commercially used probe test (PACE 2, Gen-Probe Inc, USA) has been developed using DNA–RNA hybridization to increase sensitivity for detecting chlamydial RNA. This molecular test is relatively specific and demonstrates sensitivity similar to both antigen detection and cell culture methods.[6,7]

Molecular DNA and RNA tests are becoming the best tests for the diagnosis of *C. trachomatis* genital infections, since both demonstrate high sensitivity and specificity, and can be used for examining a large range of specimens, including vulvovaginal swabs and first voided urine (FVU).[3,6] During the last two decades, several molecular tests have been introduced for diagnosis of *C. trachomatis* genital infections. These include classical PCR, real-time PCR (Roche Diagnostics, Abbott, IL, USA), ligase chain reaction LCx assay (Abbott Laboratories, USA), transcription-mediated amplification (Gen Probe), and nucleic acid sequence-based amplification (bioMerieux, Nancy L'Etoile, France).[9] All tests manipulate specimens according to manufacturers' specifications.[9] All molecular amplification tests are based on amplification of multiple copy genes that encode on cryptic plasmid of *C. trachomatis*, or on gene products such as rRNAs.[9] All molecular methods are highly specific bending preventing any contamination while performing the reaction. Clinical evaluations of these methods have demonstrated higher sensitivity than culture and other noncultural methods (microscopy, immunoassays).[6,9] There is still ongoing research directed to improve the diagnosis of all bacterial STIs using multiplex PCR, particularly DNA microarray method.

Mycoplasma species

These are the smallest free-living organisms grown on special culture media. *M. genitalium* has the smallest genome of all *Mycoplasma* species. The importance of *M. genitalium* in causing human disease, and especially genital tract disease, was recognized after the introduction of PCR technology.[10] There is strong evidence that *M. genitalium* causes nonspecific urethritis in men, but there is still not enough evidence to confirm that presence of this bacterium is commonly associated with epididymitis and prostatitis and may cause infertility.[3,11,12] In addition, *M. genitalium* has emerged in recent years as a sexually transmitted pathogen causing, in women, cervicitis, PID, and infertility.[13]

Laboratory Diagnosis

M. genitalium has fastidious growth requirements; it needs special culture medium. The organism grows slowly over a few weeks before it can be identified in culture.[14,15] Serological tests can be used in epidemiological studies but have shown limited importance in diagnosis of acute clinical cases,[16] while molecular tests are useful for detection of clinical disease caused by *M. genitalium*. However, because of the presence of a few mycoplasmas in some infected patients, molecular tests may have limited value, and there is still no commercially available test used for rapid diagnostic purposes.[11,14]

Ureaplasma Species

U. urealyticum is a part of the *Mycoplasma* group. The organism is considered a commensal in the lower genitourinary tract of sexually active men and women.[17] Ureaplasmal infection in men is found to be associated with urethritis, prostatitis, and epididymitis, whereas, in women, it may cause endometritis, chorioamnionitis, spontaneous abortion, and prematurity/low birth weight. Additionally, the organism may cause complications presented as arthritis and urinary calculi in susceptible adults.[18–20] Recent studies recommend division of *U. urealyticum* into two new species: *U. parvum* and *U. urealyticum* The actual role of *U. urealyticum* in males in causing chronic genital disease, and infertility remains a controversial issue similar to the infection with *M. genitalium*.[17,20]

Laboratory Diagnosis

Ureaplasmal infections can be diagnosed by culture; its culture requires 2–5 days, whereas molecular assays can detect their infections in few hours.[19] PCR-based methods have recently replaced conventional culture to detect ureaplasmas in clinical specimens and can help in discrimination between the two common *Ureaplasma* species.[21] Classic microbiological culture methods are much less sensitive than PCR; less than half of the PCR positive tests in semen, urine, prostatic secretion, cervical swab, amniotic fluid, and vaginal specimen indicated a positive culture.[22,23] In 1992, for the first time, PCR method was used for detection of human ureaplasmas in clinical samples;[17] after that, PCR methods have been increasingly introduced in the diagnosis of Ureaplasma infections.[3,17] Only well-designed PCR tests can detect the two *Ureaplasma spp.*, and for this reason, most previous studies have failed to discriminate between the *Ureaplasma spp.*[17] To detect species of ureaplasmas subunits, urease gene should be included along with 16S rRNA genes and the multiple-banded antigen gene (MBA).[22,23] Ureaplasma species can be identified at the serovar level by PCR; specific genotyping primers are available for partial serovar identification.[21] By applying a combination of sequencing and restriction enzyme analysis, Ureaplasma serovars and subtypes can be successfully determined.[21]

Application of quantitative PCR methods and PCR serotyping can help to discriminate between harmless commensal colonization and clinically significant ureaplasma infection.[17,21,23] Real-time TaqMan PCR methods have been recognized to allow quantitative detection of ureaplasma infection rapidly, specifically and with high sensitivity compared to conventional PCR, using the same primer sets and cycling conditions.[17,23] Accurate differentiation between *U. parvum*, *U. urealyticum,* and other serovars can be done with real-time TaqMan PCR or traditional PCR methods.[3,17]

TABLE 13.1 Primers Sequence Used for the Detection of *C. trachomatis,*
U. urealyticum, and M. genitalium

Pathogenic Bacteria	Primers	Primers Sequence 5'-3'	Target Gene	Size (bp)[a]
C. trachomatis	Forward Reverse	5'-CTAGGCGTTTGTACTCCGTCA 5'-TCCTCAGGAGTTTATGCACT	Orf8	200
M. genitalium	Forward Reverse	5'AGTTGATGAAACCTTAACCCCTTG 5'CATTACCAGTTAAACCAAAGCCT	Mgpa	346
U. urealyticum	UMS 170 UMA263	5'-GAAACGACGTCCATAAGCAACT 5'GCAATCTGCTCGTGAAGTATTAC	UreA-B	423
U. parvum	UMS 57 UMA 222	5TTAAATCTTAGTGTTCATATTTTTAC 5T-GTAAGTGCAGCATTAAATTCAATG		326

[a]Base pair.

Table 13.1 shows all the mostly used specific primers for detection of these fastidious STD agents.

In conclusion, there is still a need to develop more easily specific molecular methods for the detection of these fastidious and potential causative agents of sexually transmitted diseases.

QUESTIONS

1. Serological tests can be used for the diagnosis of nonspecific urethristis caused by:
   (a) *Chlamydia trachomati*
   (b) *Neisssseria gonorrhea*
   (c) *Ureaplasma urealyticum*
   (d) *Mycoplasm genitalium*
   (e) None of the above
2. Which of the following is associated with *Chlamydia trachomatis* infection in women?
   (a) Asymptomatic infection
   (b) Can be rapidly diagnosed using MaCoy culture
   (c) Heavy urethral pus discharge
   (d) Both (a) and (b)
   (e) None of the above
3. Nonspecific urethristis is commonly caused by:
   (a) *Chlamydia trachomatis*
   (b) *Mycoplasma hominis*
   (c) *Neisssseria gonorrhea*
   (d) Both (a) and (b)
   (e) Both (b) and (c)
4. *Mycoplasma genitalium* may cause the following in men:
   (a) Epididymitis
   (b) Prostatitis
   (c) Infertility
   (d) Both (a) and (b)
   (e) All of the above

5. *Chlamydia trachomatis* infection can be rapidly detected using PCR on the following:
   (a) Fresh urine
   (b) High-vulvovaginal swab
   (c) Urethral discharge
   (d) Both (a) and (b)
   (e) All of the above

REFERENCES

1. Newman L, Rowley J, Vander Hoorn S, et al. Global estimates of the prevalence and incidence of four curable sexually transmitted infections in 2012 Based on systematic review and global reporting. *PLoS One.* 2015;10(12):e0143304.
2. World Health Organization, Department of Reproductive Health Research. *Global Incidence and Prevalence of Selected Curable Sexually Transmitted Infections.* Geneva, Switzerland: 2012.
3. Abusarah AE, Awwad MZ, Charvalos E, Shehabi AA. Molecular detection of potential sexually transmitted pathogens in semen and urine specimens of infertile and fertile males. *Diag Microbiol Infect Dis.* 2013;77: 283–286.
4. Gdoura R, Kchaou W, Ammar-Keskes L, et al. Assessment of *Chlamydia trachomatis, Ureaplasma urealyticum, Ureaplasma parvum, Mycoplasma hominis, and Mycoplasma genitalium* in semen and first void urine specimens of asymptomatic male partners of infertile couples. *J Androl.* 2008;29(2):198-206.
5. Esen B, Gozalan A, Sevindi DF, et al. *Ureaplasma urealyticum*: presence among sexually transmitted diseases. *Jpn J Infect Dis.* 2016 Mar 18.
6. Bebear C, de Barbeyrac B. Genital *Chlamydia trachomatis* infections. *Clin Microbiol Infect.* 2009;15(1):4–10.
7. Carey AJ, Beagley KW. *Chlamydia trachomatis*, a hidden epidemic: effects on female reproduction and options for treatment. *Am J Reprod Immunol.* 2010;63(6):576–586.
8. Kapoor S. Re-emergence of lymphogranuluma vererum. *J Eur Acad Dermatol Venereology.* 2008;22 (4): 409–416.
9. Chernesky MA. The laboratory diagnosis of *Chlamydia trachomatis* infections. *Can J Infect Dis Med Microbiol.* 2005;16(1):39–44.
10. Daley GM, Russell DB, Tabrizi SN, McBride J. *Mycoplasma genitalium*: a review. *Int J STD AIDS.* 2014;25(7):475-487.
11. Shehabi AA, Awwad Z, Al-Ramahi M, Abu-Qatouseh L, Charvalos E. Diagnosis of *Mycoplasma genitalium* and *Trichomonas vaginalis* in Jordanian patients attending university hospital. *Am J Infect Dis.* 2009;5(1):7–10.
12. Weinstein SA, Stiles BG. A review of the epidemiology, diagnosis and evidence-based management of *Mycoplasma genitalium. Sex Health.* 2011; 8(2):143–158.
13. McGowin CL, Anderson-Smits C. *Mycoplasma genitalium*: an emerging cause of sexually transmitted disease in women. *PLoS Pathog.* 2011;7(5):e1001324.
14. Shipitsyna E, Savicheva A, Solokovskiy E, et al. Guidelines for the laboratory diagnosis of *Mycoplasma genitalium* infections in East European countries. *Acta Derm Venereol.* 2010;90(5):461–467.
15. Ross JD, Jensen JS. *Mycoplasma genitalium* as a sexually transmitted infection: implications for screening, testing, and treatment. *Sex Transm Infect.* 2006;82(4):269–271.
16. Jensen JS. *Mycoplasma genitalium* infections. Diagnosis, clinical aspects, and pathogenesis. *Dan Med Bull.* 2006;53(1):1–27.
17. Juhász E, Ostorházib E, Pónyaib K, Sillo P, Párduczc L, Rozgonyib F. Ureaplasmas: from commensal flora to serious infections. *Rev Med Microbiol.* 2011;22:73–83.
18. Zhang ZH, Zhang HG, Dong Y, Han RR, Dai RL, Liu RZ. *Ureaplasma urealyticum* in male infertility in Jilin Province, North-east China, and its relationship with sperm morphology. *J Int Med Res.* 2011;39(1):33–40.
19. Zeighami H, Peerayeh SN, Yazdi RS, Sorouri R. Prevalence of *Ureaplasma urealyticum* and *Ureaplasma parvum* in semen of infertile and healthy men. *Int J STD AIDS.* 2009;20(6):387–390.
20. Volgmann T, Ohlinger R, Panzig B. *Ureaplasma urealyticum*: harmless commensal or underestimated enemy of human reproduction? A review. *Arch Gynecol Obstet.* 2005;273:133–139.

21. Xiao L, Glass J I, Paralanov V, et al. Detection and characterization of human Ureaplasma species and serovars by real-time PCR. *J Clin Microbiol.* 2010;48(8):2715–2723.

22. Wang Y, Liang C, Wu J, Xu C, Qin S, Gao E. *Ureaplasma urealyticum* infections in the genital tract affect semen quality? *Asian J Androl.* 2006;8(5):562–568.

23. Waites KB, Katz B, Schelonka RL. Mycoplasmas and Ureaplasmas as neonatal pathogens. *Clin Microbiol Rev.* 2005;18(4):757–789.